Chest Drains in Daily Clinical Practice

Thomas Kiefer

Editor

Chest Drains in Daily Clinical Practice

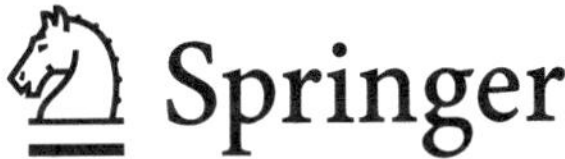 Springer

Editor
Thomas Kiefer
Lungenzentrum Bodensee
Klinikum Konstanz
Konstanz
Germany

ISBN 978-3-319-32338-1   ISBN 978-3-319-32339-8   (eBook)
DOI 10.1007/978-3-319-32339-8

Library of Congress Control Number: 2016958757

Printed on acid-free paper

This Springer imprint is published by Springer Nature
The registered company is Springer International Publishing AG
The registered company address is: Gewerbestrasse 11, 6330 Cham, Switzerland

To Gerlinde and Julia

Preface

This book is addressed to all professions who have to deal with chest drains – not only physicians of any specialisation but also nurses. It is my strong conviction that – with the exception of very few – all who work in somatic acute and emergency medicine should be able to manage chest drains and chest drain systems properly!

This is so important because a chest drain managed in the wrong way can be truly dangerous or even life threatening for the patient.

According to my knowledge, so far there is no such an elaborated book dealing with chest drains and chest drain systems covering all issues – beginning with anatomy and ending up with pain management and physiotherapy. That's why I am very grateful that the publishing company Springer made this project possible. I also want to thank my co-authors, who made it happened and helped publish this book just on schedule due to their tremendous work. My special thanks concerning this English edition of the text book go to Dr. Sarah Counts from Yale University who transformed my "school English" into a readable textbook!

Those who will read the entire book will mention that there are some reiterations concerning one or more chapters. This is intended! On the one hand it may make sense to repeat important aspects from a didactic point of view. On the other hand, the more experienced reader will pick just the chapter they are interested in.

I am open to critics and would appreciate to receive critics because this is the only way to improve and which hopefully may lead to a second edition!

Konstanz, September 2016

Contents

Contributors

Stefano Cafarotti Chirurgia toracica EOC, Ospedale San Giovanni, Bellinzona, Switzerland

Adalgisa Condoluci Chirurgia toracica EOC, Ospedale San Giovanni, Bellinzona, Switzerland

Sarah Counts Cardiothoracic Surgery, Yale School Medicine, New Haven, CT, USA

Peter Ehrhardt Klinik für Unfallchirurgie, Orthopädie und Handchirurgie, Klinikum Konstanz, Gesundheitsverbund Landkreis Konstanz, Konstanz, Germany

Fabian Graeb Karl-Olga-Krankenhaus ICU, Stuttgart, Germany

Erich Hecker Klinik für Thoraxchirurgie, Ev. Krankenhausgemeinschaft Herne, Castrop-Rauxel gGmbH, Herne, Germany

Rolf Inderbitzi Chirurgia toracica EOC, Ospedale San Giovanni, Bellinzona, Switzerland

Thomas Kiefer Klinik für Thoraxchirurgie, Lungenzentrum Bodensee, Klinikum Konstanz, Konstanz, Germany

Christian Kugler Klinik für Thoraxchirurgie, Lungen Clinic Grosshansdorf GmbH, Großhansdorf, Germany

Dana Mergner Sektionsleiterin Schmerztherapie, Klinikum Konstanz, Konstanz, Germany

Kathrin Süss Asklepios Fachkliniken München-Gauting, Gauting, Germany

Jan Volmerig Klinik für Thoraxchirurgie, Ev. Krankenhausgemeins chaft Herne, Castrop-Rauxel gGmbH, Herne, Germany

Chapter 1
Anatomy of the Chest Wall and the Pleura

Peter Ehrhardt

1.1 Introduction

The chest wall represents the outer covering of the chest and shelters the organs inside the thorax. Due to its mobility and the wall structure, which is comparable to a cage, it plays an active role in the function of breathing when the intrathoracic volume is changed. During inspiration the volume increases and during expiration it decreases, therefore generating a negative or a positive pressure respectively. According to the law of Boyle-Mariotte, gases move constantly as a result of pressure and volume.

The chest wall is construced as a cage with variable rods. The spaces within the rods are the intercostal spaces. This space has to be air tight, robust in regards to pressure, while also being adequately mobile for ventilation. This is possible with the help of the pleural space which is created by two sheets of pleura, the parietal and visceral layers. The pleural space allows the lung to slide during inspiration and expiration, keeping the lung expanded due to adhesive forces.

P. Ehrhardt
Klinik für Unfallchirurgie, Orthopädie und Handchirurgie,
Klinikum Konstanz, Gesundheitsverbund Landkreis Konstanz,
Luisenstr. 7, 78464 Konstanz, Germany
e-mail: Peter.Ehrhardt@glkn.de

© Springer International Publishing Switzerland 2017
T. Kiefer (ed.), *Chest Drains in Daily Clinical Practice*,
DOI 10.1007/978-3-319-32339-8_1

1.2   The Compostion and Margins of the Chest Wall

The sternum and cartilage of ribs 1–10 represent the anterior chest wall. The posterior part consists of 12 thoracic vertebrae and the posterior aspects of ribs 1–12. Laterally the chest cavity consists of ribs 1–12.

The thoracic aperture is created by the first ribs, the first thoracic vertebra, the upper edge of the sternum, the nerves, and the blood vessels, which together with the trachea and esophagus compose the upper opening of the chest.

The lower chest aperture is much wider and is formed by the costal arch, the free ribs (11th and 12th), and the sternum. The costal arches form an angle called the *Angulus infrasternalis* (epigastric angle) that opens caudally. This varies according to age, sex, and body compostion. In infants and women it is typically wider as compared to men (70°).

The diaphragm seals the lower chest aperture. Due to the negative pressure inside the pleural space, it is sucked cranially creating a dome.

The space between two ribs is called the intercostal space. The space is strengthened with muscles and ligaments which prevent sinking during inspiration. This whole construction is called the chest wall.

Anatomical regions are defined by the chest wall's surface:

Ventral: *Regio pectoralis / mammaria, Regio infraclavicularis, Regio parasternalis, Regio hypchondriaca*

Lateral: *Regio axillaris*

Dorsal: *Regio suprascapularis, Regios scapularis, Regio infrascapularis*

Orientation during a clinical examination and/or therapeutic procedure can be done with the assistance of anatomical lines: (Figs. 1.1 and 1.8)

- *Linea sternalis*
- *Linea parasternalis*
- *Linea medioclavicularis (MCL)*
- *Linea axillaris anterior, media, posterior*
- *Linea scapularis*
- *Linea paravertebralis*

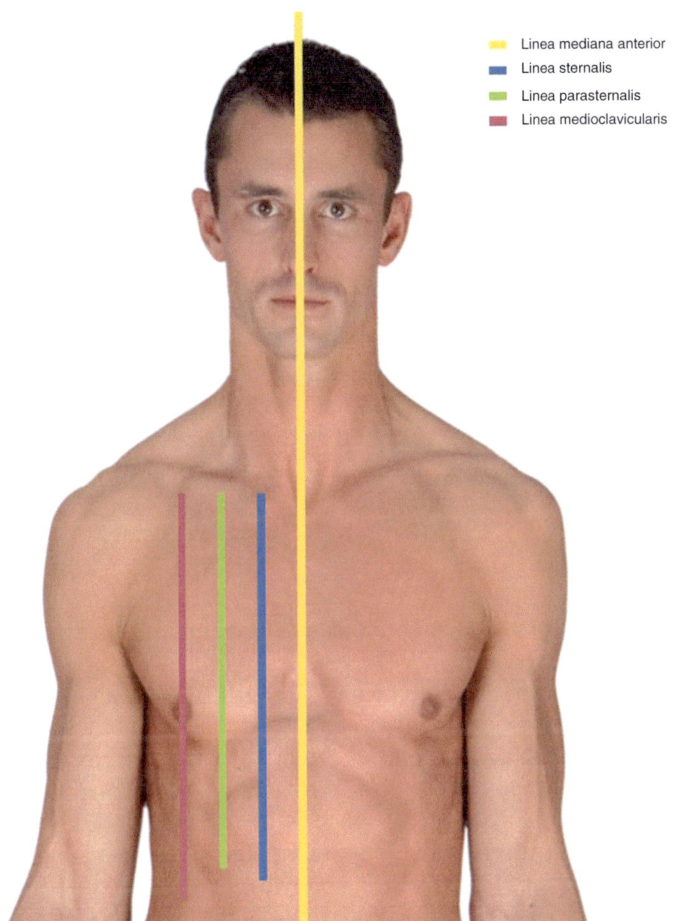

FIGURE 1.1 Anatomical lines of the anterior chest wall (Tilmann BN (2010), Ventrale Rumpfwand. In: Anatomie, Springer-Verlag Berlin Heidelberg, S. 816, Abb. 21.1)

Certain ribs and intercostal spaces can be located by palpating these structures.

The margin between the corpus and manubrium sterni is called the angulus sterni (Ludovici or sternal angle) which is visible and located next to the second rib. The first ribs cannot be palpated as they are covered by the clavicles. The second ribs and below can be identified.

1.3   Bony Components and Joints

The sternum consists of the manubrium sterni, the corpus sterni, and the processus xiphoideus. The manubrium is linked with the clavicles on each side and also with the first ribs with the help of cartilagenous joints, called synchondroses. Ribs 2–7 articulate laterally at the corpus sterni. The xiphoid is not attached to any ribs.

In general, the ribs in humans are numbered the same as their corresponding vertebral bodies. There are 12 pairs of ribs with some of them rudimentary and fused with the vertebral bodies in so called rib stumps.

The ribs are divided into real ribs (costae verae, 1–7) that have sternal joints, false ribs (costae spuriae, 8–10) with cartilagenous joints to the costal arch (arcus costalis), and free ribs (costae fluctuantes, 11–12) that end in the soft tissue of the lateral chest wall. The 12th rib is not always present.

The head of the rib (caput costae) articulates laterally with the vertebral body and there is a second articulation between the transverse process and the vertebral body. The rib neck is located between these articulations and acts as the longitudinal axis for rib movement. The neck of the rib is followed by the body of the rib (collum costae), turning anteriorly at an angle (angulus costae). Anteriorly all bony tissue is followed by cartilage which represents the elastic link with the sternum (Fig. 1.2).

The ribs move upwards during inspiration around their rib neck and downwards during expiration. This volume increase and decrease is due to changes in both the sagital and transverse directions. The mobility of the chest is guaranteed by the joints between the vertebral bodies and ribs as well as by the interactions between the cartilage, sternum, and costal arch.

The costosternal complex moves cranially and ventrally (sagittal extension). The lower ribs move towards cranially and laterally to increase the diameter of the chest in the transverse direction (Fig. 1.3).

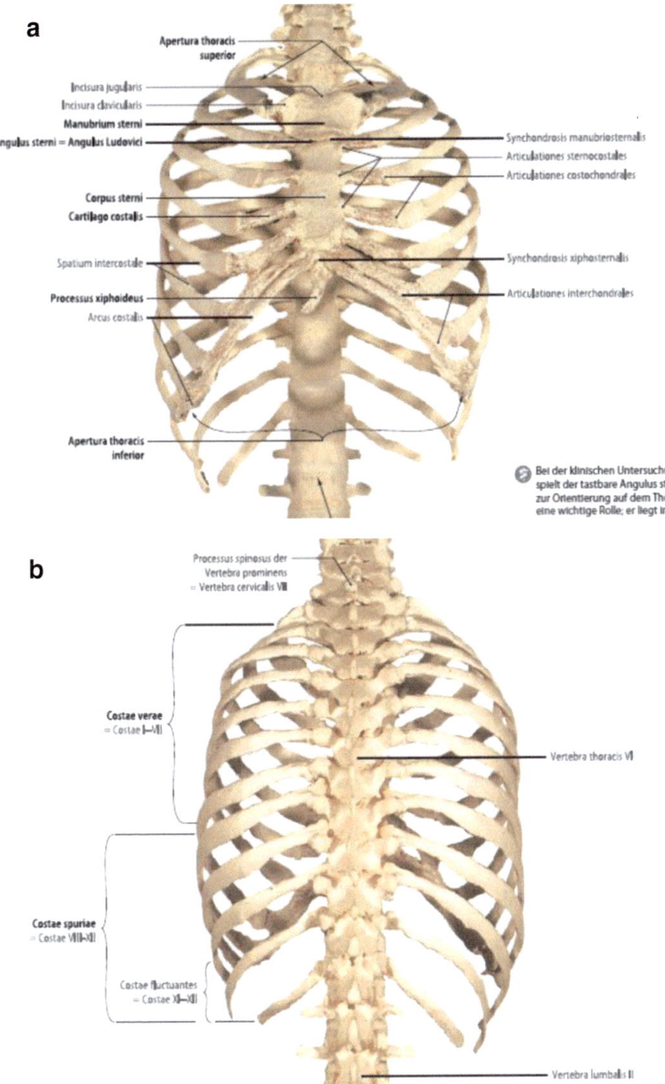

FIGURE 1.2 Bony chest (**a**) view from anterior, (**b**) view from posterior (Tilmann BN (2005), Rumpfskelett In: Atlas der Anatomie, Springer-Verlag Berlin Heidelberg, S. 187/188, Abb. 4.1, 4.2. (jeweils oberer Abschnitt ohne Becken))

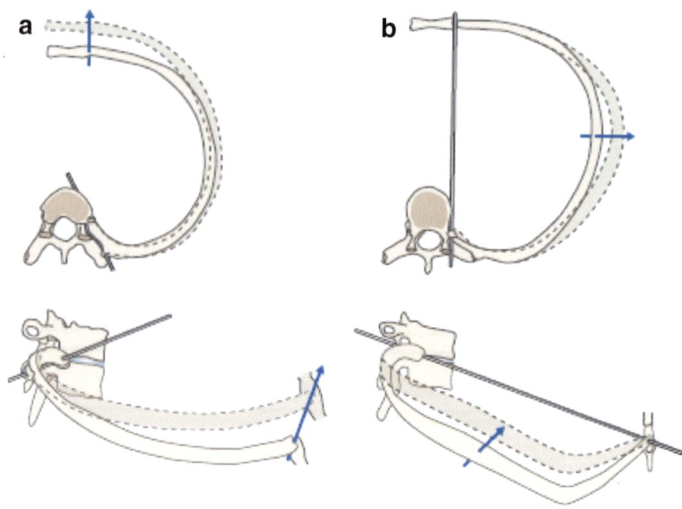

FIGURE 1.3 Movement of the ribs during inspiration and expiration (van Gestel A et al. (2010), Atembewegungsapparat. In: Physiotherapie bei chronischen Atemwegs- und Lungenerkrankungen, Springer-Verlag Berlin Heidelberg, S. 17, Abb. 2.2)

At the lower edge of the rib, the sulcus costaeis is located where the intercostal vessels and the intercostal nerve run. The intercostal muscles are attached to the edges of the ribs (Fig. 1.9).

1.4   Muscles of the Chest Wall

The lung itself does not have any muscles and therefore the muscles of the chest wall and diaphragm are responsible for the movements that let us breathe. Some of the chest wall muscles can be used as helpful anatomical landmarks.

At the neck, the chest is attached by the three scalene muscles, the intercostal muscles, and the muscles eminating from ribs 1 and 2 to the vertebral bodies (1–7). They are responsible for the flexion of the upper spine anteriorly and for lifting the ribs during inspiration (Fig. 1.4).

The Pectoralis major muscle covers the upper and lateral part of the chestwall like a shelf and creates the outline of the

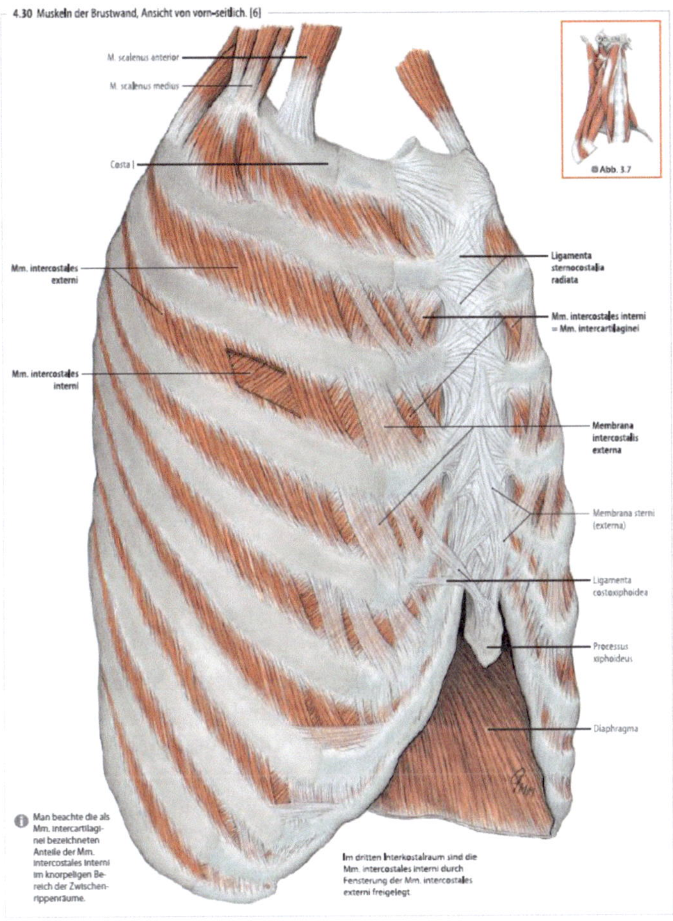

FIGURE 1.4 Chestwall muscles, view from anterolateral (Tilmann BN (2005), Muskeln der Brustwand. In: Atlas der Anatomie, Springer-Verlag Berlin Heidelberg, S. 204, Abb. 4.30 (jeweils oberer Abschnitt ohne Becken))

chestwall. It originates from the medial clavicle, the sternum, the cartilages of ribs 5–7, as well as from the rectus sheath, and inserts at the tuberculum majus humeri. The lower edge of the muscle creates the anterior axillary plication. This muscle causes a strong adduction and rotation of the arm and its lower portion acts as an auxillary breathing muscle.

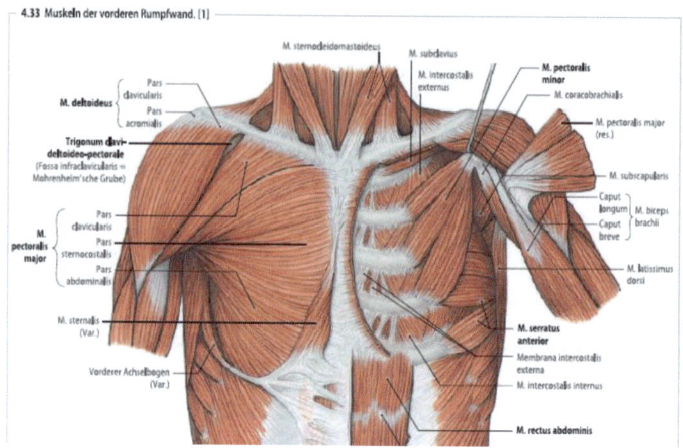

FIGURE 1.5 Muscles of the anterior chestwall (Tilmann BN (2005), Muskeln der Brustwand. In: Atlas der Anatomie, Springer-Verlag Berlin Heidelberg, S. 207, Abb. 4.33 (oberer Abschnitt))

The Pectoralis minor muscle is completely covered by the Pectoralis major muscle. It derives from the ribs 3–5 and connects to the processus coracoideus of the shoulder. This muscle pulls the shoulder anteriorly and downwards and also lifts the chest as an auxillary breathing muscle (Fig. 1.5).

The intercostal muscles consist of two layers of short muscles between the ribs oriented in different directions. The more external layer is made of the *intercostales externi* muscle which is oriented craniolaterally to mediocaudally from the lower edge of the upper rib to the upper edge of the rib below. The *intercostales interni* muscle is located underneath oriented opposite of the externi and therefore from craniomedial to laterocaudal. Both muscles help to maintain the appropriate tension of the rib cage. The outer muscles lift the chest up (inspiration) and the inner ones lower it and strengthen expiration.

A soft tissue layer allows room for the intercostal vessels and nerve and separates the *intercostales interni muscles* from the *intercostales intimi muscles.* These muscle fibers are oriented in the same direction. The *intercostales interni*

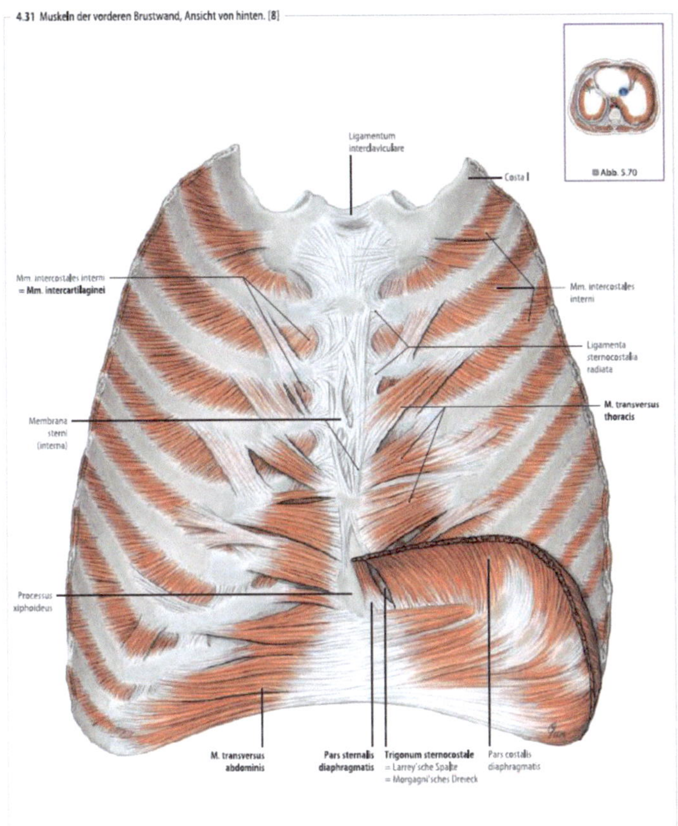

FIGURE 1.6 Muscles of the anterior chest wall – view from behind (Tilmann BN (2005), Muskeln der Brustwand. In: Atlas der Anatomie, Springer-Verlag Berlin Heidelberg, S. 205, Abb. 4.31)

muscles that create a longer layer of muscle going over the first and second rib are called *Subcostales muscles.*

Muscles running transversely from the inner surface of the sternum towards the ribs are called the *transversus thoracis muscles* (Fig. 1.6).

The lower border of the chest cavity made up of the diaphragm which originates from the lower chest aperture and the vertebral bodies 1–4 of the lumbar column. The

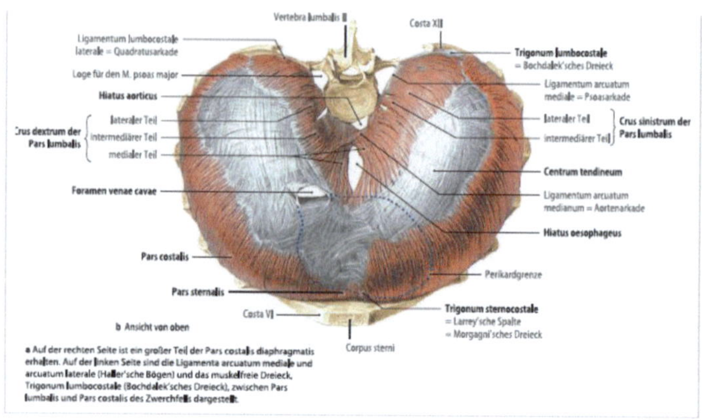

FIGURE 1.7 Diaphragm, view from above (Tilmann BN (2005), Hintere Rumpfwand. In: Atlas der Anatomie, Springer-Verlag Berlin Heidelberg, S. 212, Abb. 4.40b)

diaphragm is a muscle measuring 3–5 mm thick which creates a dome with a tendon in the center. In regard to surface area it is the largest muscle in the human body. Due to the elastic recoil of the lung which is transferred throughout the pleural cavity, the diaphragm lifts upwards creating the diaphragmatic dome which is slightly higher on the right side. The top of the dome can vary about 6–7 cm from inspiration to expiration respectively. Contraction of the diaphragmatic muscle causes it to flatten and thus increases the volume of the chest cavity (Fig. 1.7).

1.5   Topography of the Chest Cavity

The pleura is a serous skin that consists of mesothelium, a squamous epithelium (one layer), and the lamina propria. The pleura covers the lung and chest wall. There are two layers called the visceral pleura and the parietal pleura which are separated by a capillary gap filled up with 2–4 ml of fluid. This configuration allows the lung to slide up and down and, despite the elastic recoil, keeps the lung expanded.

In the pleural cavity there is a negative pressure due to the elastic recoil of the lung fighting against the adhesive forces generated by the pleural fluid. These forces during inspiration pull the lung to follow the chest wall.

The visceral pleura covers the entire lung with the exception of the hilar region. The parietal pleura covers the inner chest wall similar to wallpaper. The regions where the parietal pleura covers the mediastinum, chest wall, or diaphragm are correspondingly named *Pars mediastinalis, Pars costalis* and *Pars diaphragmatica.* Both of the pleural cavities are closed spaces completely filled with the lungs without any connection to each other, the atmosphere, or the other lung. The shape of the pleural cavity is determined by the lordosis of the vertebral column. The domes of the diaphragm create an optimal shape for expansion of the volume of the chest cavity during inspiration. In the middle, the two pleural cavities are separated by the mediastinum anteriorly and vertebral collum posteriorly. At the middle aspect of the sternum, the two pleural cavities are separated by the parietal pleura which are separated by the parietal pleura and are in contact with each other.

Cranially the pleural cavity extends for 2–3 cm above the upper chest aperture (*Cupula pleurae*).

The pleura cavities have narrow spaces called *Recessus pleurales* where the lung can expand which are located anteriorly between the chest wall and sternum and laterally between diaphragm and chest wall. The *recessus costomediastinalis* on the left side between pericardium and chestwall is somewhat wider as compared to the right side. The *recessus costodiaphragmaticus* creates an additional deep semicircular space reaching nearly to the origin of the diaphragm (Fig. 1.8).

In the back, the recessus may extend up to 2 cm below the 12th rib therefore putting it in the neighborhood of the right lobe of the liver and on the left towards the stomach, spleen, and upper pole of the kidney (Fig. 1.8, Table 1.1). The margins of the lung shift during inspiration and expiration anteriorly for 1–2 cm and in the back for 5–6 cm. Normally the lower margin of the right lung is 1–2 cm above the lung margin on the left side.

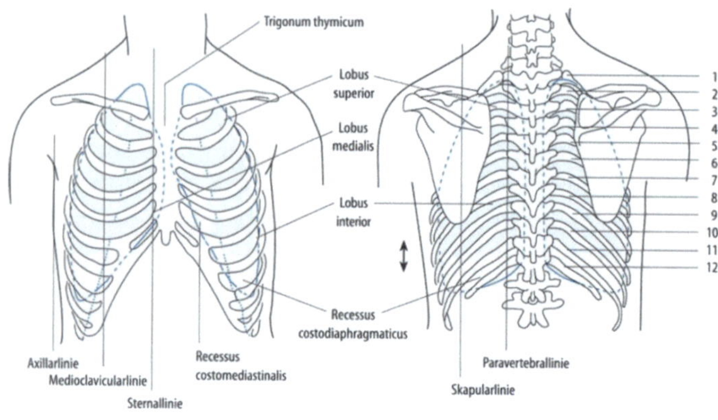

FIGURE 1.8 Margins of the lung and the pleura (Larsen R et al. (2004), Anatomie der Atmungsorgane. In: Beatmung, Springer-Verlag Berlin Heidelberg, S. 16, Abb. 1.9)

TABLE 1.1 Margins of the lung and pleura as projected on the chest-wall during resting expiratory position [2]

	Sternal line	Mid clavicular line	Mid axillary lini	Paravertebral line
Margin of the plaura	6th rib	7th rib	9th rib	12th rib ≙ 12th DP
Margin of the lung	6th rib	6th rib	8th rib	11th rib ≙ 10th DP

[a]DP = dorsal process

There are projections on the bony chest wall of the fissures (in resting expiratory position):

The fissure between left upper and lower lobe *(Fissura obliqua)* is at the level of the fourth rib posteriorly and the third dorsal process respectively and sinks down anteriorly to the cartilagenous junction of the sixth rib with the sternum.

On the right side, the horizontal fissure between the upper and lower lobe is located above the fourth rib in the axillary line heading towards the sternum and the oblique fissure

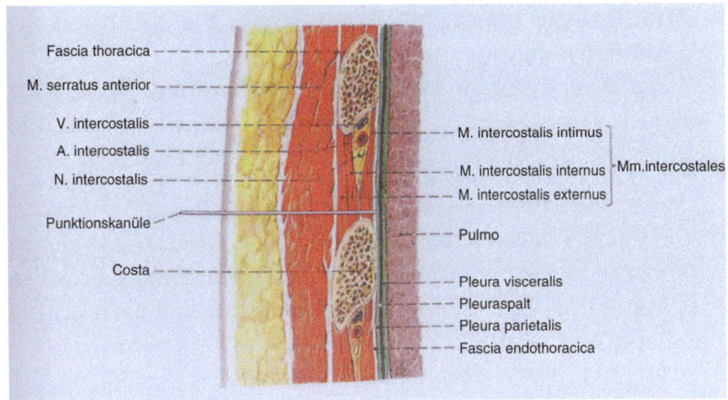

FIGURE 1.9 Upright section through the posterior chest wall at the level of the posterior axillary line (Christ B. (2003) Skelett- und Muskelsystem. In: Drenckhahn D (Hrsg) Anatomie Band 1, 16. Aufl. Urban & Fischer Verlag München Jena with permission from Drenckhahn, Benninghoff, Anatomie Band 1, 17.Auflage 2008 © Elsevier GmbH, Urban & Fischer, München)

going down to the sixth rib. In between these two is the location of the middle lobe [3].

The innervation of the costal pleura is provided by the corresponding intercostsal nerve and the mediastinal and diaphragmatic pleurae by the phrenic nerve. These nerves have a lot of pain fibers. Pain is noticed as an acute stabbing pain and can be localized precisely.

1.6   Layers of the Chest wall

The anterior and lateral parts of the chestwall in particular are easily accessible for invasive procedures. Therefore a deep knowledge the anatomy is mandatory. Three layers can be described:

- **Superficial layer** consisting of skin, subcutaneous soft and fatty tissue (including the mammary gland, which is attached via the membrana sterni with the sternum. Fig. 1.9).

- ***Middle layer*** consisting of muscles of the chest and the abdomen including their fascias
- ***Deep layer*** consisting of the skeleton, intercostal muscles, blood vessels/nerves, *fascia endothoracica* (covers the inner surface of the chest wall), and parietal pleura.

The *Fascia endothoracica* lies in between the inner muscles of the chest wall and the *pars costalis* of the parietal pleura which both are very strongly combined. In a cranial direction it continues as the fascia of the neck and caudally it covers the diaphragm.

1.7   Nerve and Blood Supply

Innervation of the chest wall is mainly supplied by the inter-costal nerves (intercostales nerves) which derive from the spinal cord at each segmental level as rami anteriores. They run along the lower edge of the ribs. They supply the intercostal muscles as well as the skin. In addition there are fibers that go to the perspiratory glands.

Blood supply of the chest wall is caried out by the intercostal arteries (intercostales arteries) and by the internal mammary artery (thoracica interna artery) which create a ring of vasculature in the region of the anterior chest wall.

Intercostal arteries 3–11 are directly derive from the aorta whereas arteries 1–2 derive from the truncus costocervicales. They all run along the lower edge of the ribs and anastomose with the Rr. intercostales anteriores anteriores which derive from the internal mammary artery.

Intercostal veins run together with the arteries and drain into the azygos vein posteriorly and anteriorly into internal mammary vein into the subclavian vein.

At the lower edge of the ribs, the structures are found in the following order: vein, artery, and nerve (Fig. 1.10).

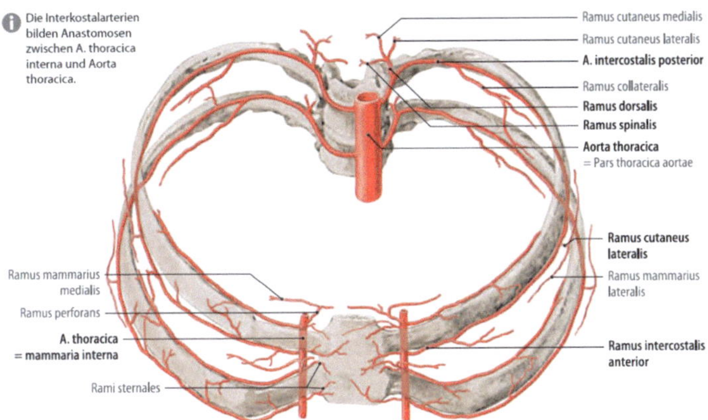

FIGURE 1.10 Arterial blood supply of the chestwall (Tilmann BN (2005), Rücken- und Nackenmuskeln. In: Atlas der Anatomie, Springer-Verlag Berlin Heidelberg, S. 218, Abb. 4.49)

Literature

1. Drenckhahn D, Benninghoff WJ (HRSG). Anatomie Band 1, 17. Aufl. Elevier GmbH, Urban & Fischer, München; 2008.
2. Duncker HR, Kummer W. Atemsystem. In: Drenckhahn D (Editor) Anatomie Band 1, 16. Aufl. Urban & Fischer Verlag München Jena; 2003.
3. Larsen B. et al. Anatomie der Atmungsorgane. In: Larsen B (Editor) Beatmung. Berlin Heidelberg: Springer; 2004.
4. Roberts KP, Weinhaus AJ. Vessels oft he thoracic wall. In: Iaizzo PA (Editor) Handbook of cardiac anatomy, physiology and devices. Totowa: Humana Press Inc; 2005.
5. Tillmann BN. Atlas der Anatomie, Springer Heidelberg; 2005.
6. Tillmann BN. Ventrale Rumpfwand. In: Zilles K, Tillmann BN (Editor), Anatomie, Springer Heidelberg, Berlin; 2010.
7. Van Gestel AJR, Teschler H. Physiotherapie bei chronischen Atemwegserkrankungen. Springer Berlin, Heidelberg; 2010.

Chapter 2
Physiology and Pathophysiology of the Pleura

Stefano Cafarotti, Adalgisa Condoluci, and Rolf Inderbitzi

2.1 Introduction

The physiology and pathophysiology of the pleural space can be explained simply and reasonable by reviewing the functional and anatomic composition of the pleura. The pleura represents the connection between the lung and chest wall and acts as a crucial component for breathing mechanics. The pressure present in between the two pleura sheets is also important for the physiology and pathophysiology of the pleural space and its organs. The pressure ratio from the outer side of the lung and heart on one side to the inner side of the chest wall on the other side is regulated by the intrapleural pressure. The lungs, heart, and chest wall are expandable. The volume of an expandable object depends on it elasticity and the difference in pressure from the inner to the outer side of the object. In the pleural cavity, the intrapleural pressure plays an important role concerning the volume of these three very important structures. The lymph located in the parietal pleura together with the intra pleural pressure are responsible for the production of the pleural fluid and its consistency.

S. Cafarotti • A. Condoluci • R. Inderbitzi (✉)
Chirurgia toracica EOC, Ospedale San Giovanni,
6500 Bellinzona, Switzerland
e-mail: Rolf.Inderbitzi@eoc.ch

© Springer International Publishing Switzerland 2017
T. Kiefer (ed.), *Chest Drains in Daily Clinical Practice*,
DOI 10.1007/978-3-319-32339-8_2

The pleural fluid creates a film of fluid between the parietal and visceral pleural sheets which is of functional importance. The quality and quantity of the pleural fluid represents the physiological or pathophysiological condition of the pleural space. The pleural fluid is also accessible for diagnostic procedures.

2.2 Functional Anatomy and Biology

2.2.1 Pleura

The pleura consists of two sheets (parietal and visceral pleura) which meet at the hilum and distally create a plication called the pulmonary ligament. The reflective surfaces of the healthy pleura (Fig. 2.1) are separated by the pleural space which is a capillary space filled with pleural fluid (5–15 ml). The fluid allows the pleural sheets to slide along each other. This fluid film, under healthy conditions, is free from air and gas. This allows for intrapleural pressure modulation according to positioning of the chest and for the sliding of the intrathoracic organs along the chest wall. The visceral pleura is 100–200 μm thick and is strongly adherent to the lung. The superficial mesothelium (covering cell layer) is made up of mesothelial cells which are connected to each other by desmosomes and have surface microvilli. There are three layers of soft tissue limited by a basal membrane. The main layer of the pleura consists of soft tissue covered by inner and outer boundary lamella. Between these two lamellas are where the vessels are found (Fig. 2.2). The inner lamella is located next to the alveolar walls and is connected with the interstitial soft tissue of the lung in the fissures. The parietal pleura is located via the endothoracic fascia next to the intercostal muscle and the ribs.

2.2.2 Vessels

The pleural vessels run in the soft tissue main layer. The blood supply of the visceral pleura is located in the area of

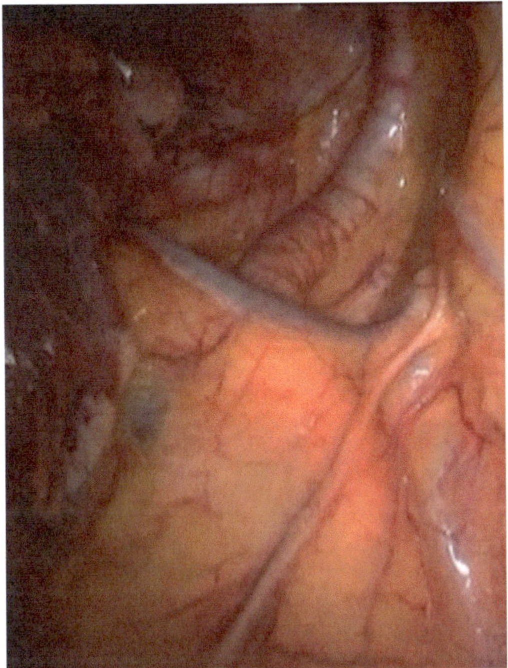

FIGURE 2.1 Normal, transparent Pleura: Left subclavian artery and phrenic nerve are visible

the ribs and the diaphragm via the pulmonary arteries and bronchial arterial branches which create anastomoses with the pulmonary arteries in all other areas. The parietal pleura is fed by the intercostal arteries in the regions of the ribs and by the *rami intercostales* of the internal mammary arteries.

2.2.3   Lymph Vessels

The lymphatics of the visceral pleura are located close to the lung in the soft tissue main layer of the pleura. Of special importance are lymphatic stomata which are 2–8 µm in diameter in the parietal pleura. In these areas the pleural space is directly connected to the draining lymphatic system [1]. The

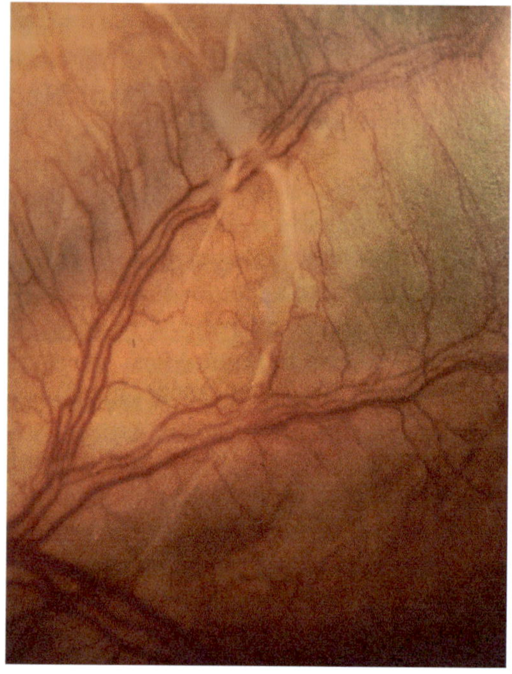

FIGURE 2.2 Layer with arterial and venous capillaries

pleural fluid circulates at a speed of 0.2 ml/kg/h, which allows for a total exchange of the fluid within one hour.

2.2.4   Mesothelium

The mesothelium is a tissue with a high metabolism that is able to produce different mediators and soluble factors for chemotactic activity and phagocytic activity. Mesothelial cells not only play an active roll in inflammatory processes but also participate in tissue repair as they synthesize collagen types I, II, and IV. Under physiologic circumstances, the pleural cell surfaces have mononuclear phagocytes that produce cytokines IL-1P, TNF-a, IL-8, and LTB-4 [3].

2.3   Physiology of the Pleural Space

2.3.1   Intrapleural Pressure

The position of the body and the phase of the breathing cycle create different pressure ratios in the pleural space. In principle a "negative pressure" is created by the elastic recoil of the lung. "Elastic recoil" is the tendency of the lung to shrink to a smaller volume than is available in the chest cavity. The lung adjusts to the significantly less elastic chest wall in regards to shape and volume in a way that the "negative" pressure is significantly higher than the elastic recoil of the lung itself. The forces that keep the lung expanded are created by the continuous evacuation of pleural fluid through the lymphatic vessels and the subpleural capillaries which prevent the intrapleural fluid from increasing. Adhesion forces between the surface of the lung and the chest wall work like a homogenous vacuum spread over the pleural surface forcing the lung to follow the chest wall during inspiration and expiration.

2.3.2   Basics in Physics [4]

The pressure (P) describes a physical condition defined for each place in space as a force being affected in all directions. Natural law (2nd law of thermodynamics) defines that the pressure between two adjacent spaces is equalized if the bounding surface allows. Negative pressure does not exist; we always look at the pressure difference (ΔP) between two different spaces (i.e. lung and pleural space). Reference pressure is the atmospheric pressure. The weight of air over the earth is 10 tons per square meter. All pressures measured in or at the human body are differences compared to the atmospheric pressure, i.e. higher or lower than the atmospheric pressure. The units of measure frequently used in medicine are listed in Table 2.1.

TABLE 2.1 Physical unit of measurement regarding pressure in medicine

	Bar	**m WS**	**Torr**	**Physical atmosphere**
	1	**1**	**1**	
	mbar	**cmH$_2$O**	**mmHg**	**1 atm**
1 atm	10^3	10^3	750	1
1 mmHg	1.3	1.3	1	$1.3*10^{-3}$
1 cmH$_2$O	1	1	0.75	10
1 mbar	1	1	0.75	10

2.3.3 *Changes in Pleural Pressure During Breathing*

Lung tissue is very elastic and is able to both increase and decrease its volume. As there is equilibrium or a pressure difference between intrapulmonary and intrapleural pressure (i.e. in atelectasis, in a pneumothorax, during single lung ventilation) the lung volume decreases from V_{tot} (2500 cm^3) to V_0 (700 cm^3). Elasticity of the lung or elastic recoil as well as the distension of the lung in the pleural cavity are responsible for the so called "negative pressure" in the pleural space. In a healthy lung with normal elastic recoil intrapleural pressure oscillates around 10 mbar.

Direct measurement of the intrapleural pressure can only be done by invasive procedures. In daily practice intrapleural pressure is determined via the esophagus, presuming that the intrapleural pressure is the same as the pressure in the esophageal area near the mediastinal pleura. The clinical relevance of the absolute measured value can be neglected.

At the end of maximal inspiration with maximal contraction of the diaphragm, a healthy adult person is able to generate a "negative" intrapleural pressure of around −200 mBar. During maximal expiration, the resistance of the abdominal musculature and the chest wall combined with a relaxed diaphragm generates an intrapleural pressure of roughly 200 mbar. In daily life, maximal values are detected during physical effort with minimal values at the end of maximal expiration which physiologically prevent atelectasis.

2.3.4   Pleural Fluid

Pleural fluid is produced by the lung interstitium, pleural capillaries, chest wall lymph vessels, and in the peritoneal cavity. Under physiological conditions, the pleural fluid is mainly derived from the capillary bed of the parietal pleura. The total amount of fluid is relatively constant during the adult lifespan. In older individuals, there is a decreased percentage of protein in the fluid and is often combined with an increased systemic blood pressure. These two factors when present together may provoke an increased production of pleural fluid leading to a visible pleural effusion [5].

The law of Starling describes the motion of fluid from the pleural capillaries to the pleural cavity. According to this law, fluids go through the vessel wall according to the effective filtration pressure (i.e. hydrostatic pressure inside minus pressure outside and colloid osmotic pressure outside minus pressure inside) and the permeability of the vessel's wall (Fig. 2.3). Under physiological conditions, there is a flow gradient from the parietal pleural capillaries to the pleural space, whereby the somewhat lower pressure in the visceral pleural capillaries leads to an outflow into the pulmonary veins rather than into the pleural cavity.

Despite the Starling mechanism, no pleural effusion develops because of the connection between the pleural space and the lymphatic system. The lymphatics in the parietal pleura drain the pleural fluid from the pleural space into the chest wall. Fluid, proteins, cells, and other components of the pleural fluid are regulated substantially by these lymphatics. Fluid filtration occurs at a speed of 0.2 ml/kg/h, which means that a 70 kg individual filtrates at a rate of 17.5 ml/h or a volume of approximately 400 ml/day. The flow rate via the lymphatics is linear with their maximum capacity for a transudate at

Abbildung 3:

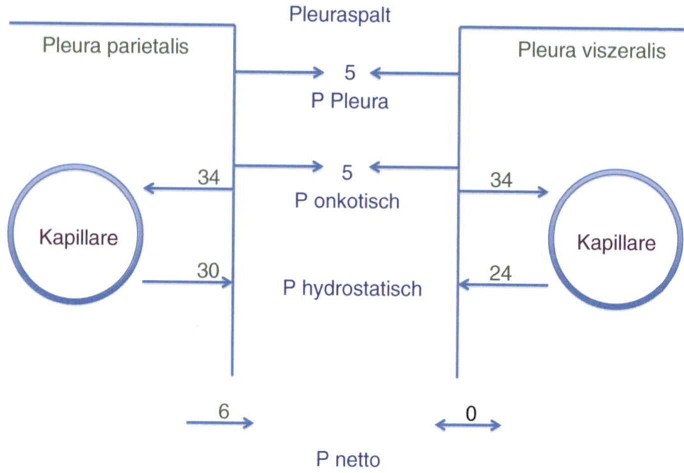

FIGURE 2.3 Pressure ratio in the pleural space: *arrows* show possible influence of pressure (in cmH$_2$O) induced by fluid movements

0.28 ml/kg/h [6]. Numerous studies have shown that exudates and fluid with protein/cells flow away mainly via the lymphatic system. Both pleural sheets are also able to directly absorb aqueous fluid due to the relatively equal osmolarity on both sides of the serosa.

2.4   Pathophysiology of the Pleural Space

2.4.1   *Air or Gas*

Air and other gases are not detectable in the pleural space under normal conditions. Either may be seen after the development of a pneumothorax due to pathologic lung changes or from an injury to the chest wall. These are not directly related to the pathophysiology of the pleural space. The development of gas in this space is an indicator of a primary or secondary infection of the pleural cavity or the pleural fluid respectively.

2.4.2   *Pleural Effusion*

A pleural effusion develops when the production of fluid exceeds fluid absorption. The main causes of increased fluid production and decreased absorption are listed in Table 2.2.

TABLE 2.2 Pathophysiologic causes leading to pleural effusion

Pathophysiology	Clinical cause
Increased intrapleural Fluid Production	
Increased intrapulmonary interstitial flow	Left heart insufficiency, Pneumonia, Pulmonary Embolism
Increased intravascular pleural pressure	Right heart insufficiency, Left heart insufficiency
Increase in intrapleural proteins	Pneumonia, Pleuritis
Decreasing intrapleural pressure	Atelectasis, Trapped lung
Decrease of pleural fluid absorption	
Obstruction of parietal lymphatic drainage (stomata)	Pleural Carcinomatosis, Pleural Empyema
Increase of systemic blood pressure	
Pathophysiology	**Clinical consequence**
Increase of hydrostatic pressure	Transsudative Effusion
Increase of vessel's permeability	Exudative Effusion

Under normal healthy conditions, fluid production into the pleural space from the parietal pleura is about 0.01 ml/kg/h. The majority of this fluid is reabsorbed by the lymphatic system of the parietal pleura at a rate up to 0.20 ml/kg/h. This means that there is a 20 fold security factor in place! [7].

The common causes of increased fluid produced from the lung interstitium include: lung edema, parapneumonic effusion, congestive heart failure, ARDS, etc. An increased intravascular pleural pressure will be followed by a pleural effusion (i.e. in right and left heart insufficiency or due to an increased concentration of proteins as seen in a hemothorax).

Conversely, a decrease in intrapleural capillary pressure, as described with the Starling law, leads to an increased fluid production in the pleura space. Typically this is the case with extensive atelectasis of a trapped lung.

There are rare conditions which overwhelm the absorptive capacity of the pleura which then lead to a pleural effusion. Examples include when there is an open connection between the chest and abdomen with ascites present or when this is an injury to the thoracic duct (i.e. chylothorax). As the parietal lymphatic drainage flows into the venous system, this increased pressure in the veins leads to backpressure and therefore to the development of a pleural effusion.

A clinically relevant pleural effusion can occur when pleural carcinomatosis obstructs the parietal lymphatic drainage. In this situation, there is usually not only the outflow obstruction but also a simultaneous increase in fluid production. A malignant pleural effusion is an indicator of advanced disease and/or the presence of pleural metastases. Pleural metastases are frequently seen with bronchogenic carcinomas (40 %) and with breast cancer (25 %). Around 10 % of malignant pleural effusions are caused by a primary pleural tumor. Mesothelioma causes greater than 90 % of these with the remainder due to CUP syndrome.

A pleural empyema represents a special form of pleural effusion. This pathophysiologic cascade occurs when there is inflammation of the pleural surface of around 200 cm^2. Initially dilatation of the vasculature causes soft tissue edema of the main layer. This is followed by a permeability disturbance leading to transudation of serious fluid and exudation of serofibrinous fluid into the pleural cavity. Pleural fibrin can lead to obstruction and also hinders evacuation via the parietal lymphatic system. Desquamation and necrosis of the mesothelium is a consequence. The typical pleural empyema involves loculated fluid chambers and a rind that develops on the pleura.

2.4.3   *Obliteration of the Pleura Space*

According to several studies, the obliteration of the pleural space leads to a more apical than basal restriction in lung function that has no clinical relevant impact [8]. The loss of fluid filtration ability after obliteration also seems to be clinically irrelevant [9]. These facts are important when considering pleurodesis, especially with young patients with spontaneous pneumothoraces.

Literature

1. Müller KM. Erkrankungen der Pleura – pathologische Anatomie, S. 325. In Nakhosteen JA, Inderbitzi R. Atlas und Lehrbuch der thorakalen Endoskopie: Bronchoskopie, Thorakoskopie. Springer Verlag; 1994.
2. Stewart PB. The rate of formation and lymphatic removal of fluid in pleural effusions. J Clin Invest. 1963;42:258–62.
3. Hausheer FH, Yabro JW. Diagnosis and treatment of malignant pleural effusion. Semin Oncol. 1985;12:54–75.
4. Linder A. Thoraxdrainagen und Drainagesysteme – Moderne Konzepte. Uni-med; 2004.
5. Broaddus VC, Araya M, Carlton DP, Bland RD. Developmental changes in pleural liquid protein concentration in sheep. Am Rev Respir Dis. 1991;143:38–41.
6. Leckie WJH, Tothill P. Albumin turnover in pleural effusion. Clin Sci. 1965;29:339–52.
7. Light RW. Parapneumonic effusions and empyema. Prc Am Thorac Soc. 2006;3:75–80.

8. Fleetham JA, Forkert L, Clarke H, Anthonisen NR. Regional lung function in the presence of pleural symphysis. Am Rev Respir Dis. 1980;122(1):33–8.
9. Wiener-Kronish JP, Broaddus VC, Albertine KH, Gropper MA, Matthay MA, Staub NC. Relationship of pleural effusions to increased permeability pulmonary edema in anesthetized sheep. J Clin Invest. 1988;82:1422–9.

Chapter 3
Indications for Draining the Chest

Christian Kugler

Inserting a chest drain may be associated with severe complications and therefore the indication for doing so must be very precise. The most important aspect in this context is the treatment goal, which has to be achieved through the procedure. Further considerations such as the type of drain (shape, diameter, and material), number of drains, and the anatomical location should align with the therapy aim. One must consider the indication for intervention in relation to the patient's clinical course. This is the only way to calculate the risk/benefit ratio of this invasive procedure.

"Draining of the Chest" addresses the "insertion of a drain in the pleural space". Drains inserted in other anatomic regions, such a mediastinum or pericardium, are excluded.

C. Kugler
Chefarzt der Klinik für Thoraxchirurgie,
LungenClinic Grosshansdorf GmbH,
Wöhrendamm 80, 22927 Großhansdorf, Germany
e-mail: c.kugler@lungenclinic.de

© Springer International Publishing Switzerland 2017
T. Kiefer (ed.), *Chest Drains in Daily Clinical Practice*,
DOI 10.1007/978-3-319-32339-8_3

3.1   General Indication Principles

3.1.1   Evacuation of Air/Gas

Air may derive from the respiratory organs (Airways, lung) themselves into the pleural space as well as from outside through the chest wall (Fig. 3.1). Perforation of the esophagus or the stomach may also be a reason for having air in the pleural space. Due to the mechanics of the diaphragm, gas may get into the pleural space from the intestines. Bacteria can produce gas in the chest cavity as well. The goal of the drain is to completely and efficiently evacuate the air from the pleural space with the intention to reexpand the lung. When the air is removed from the pleural space, it is no longer competing with lung for reexpansion. At the same time, the drain may act as a monitoring tool, showing whether there is still air coming into the pleural space or not. The

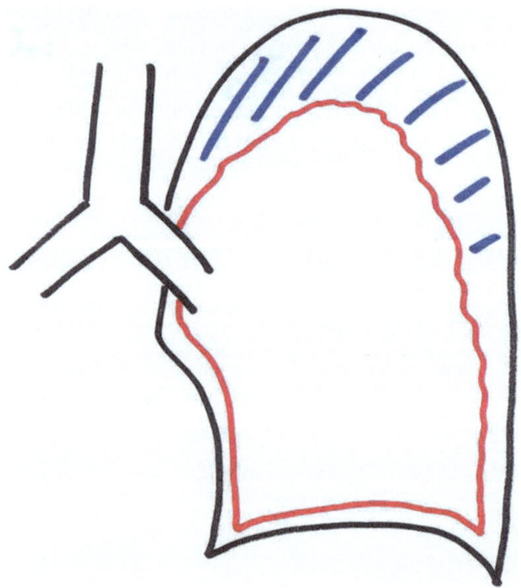

FIGURE 3.1 Aeropleura

respective drainage system utilized has to take into account that, if necessary, large amounts of air may have to be efficiently evacuated from this space with the appropriate suction capability.

With these indications in mind, the treatment goal is to restore and control the subatmospheric pressure in the pleural space after evacuating air from the pleural space. Each drainage system connected to the chest drain (Bag, Heimlich-Valve, water seal, suction device) has to fulfill this task. The indication for insertion of a chest drain may be prophylactic in some cases i.e. when there is perhaps no air in the pleural space after lung or airway surgery. The chest drain is there to monitor and treat any potential air leaks during the postoperative course of the patient. Physiologically air will accumulate mainly in the apical and anterior parts of the chest cavity. One must consider though that there are anatomical variations to consider (adhesions from the chest wall to the lung, elevation of the diaphragm, and shift of intrathoracic organs) which may allow air to accumulate in other regions of the chest cavity or multiple locations. These aspects must be taken into account as well when evaluating the indication for placing a chest drain.

3.1.2   *Evacuation of Fluids*

There are many disease states and phenomena that may cause a pleural effusion (Fig. 3.2). The simple presence of fluid in the pleural space is not an indication for a chest drain. Indications for inserting a chest drain for fluid may be the amount of fluid, the need to monitor the amount and dynamics of fluid produced, the underlying disease, to assess the quality of the fluid, prophylaxis concerning secondary effects, therapeutic considerations, and pure palliative aspects.

Fluids compete for space in relation to the lung and its expansion as was described with gas as above. Draining the fluid gives the lung its ancestral place and volume back in the confines of the chest. If the fluid shows dynamic changes such as solidification, organization or infection, this can influence the timing of intervention.

Free floating fluid in the chest cavity will accumulate mainly in the basal and posterior areas. Anatomical changes such as pleural adhesions can lead to completely different localization of the fluid, i.e. divided in several compartments (apical localization or in the fissure). These considerations need to be addressed as well as the quality of the fluid as the effectiveness of the drain can be compromised.

Preformed or secondary developed cavities in the chest cavity such as a pleuro-pulmonary mismatch after previous lung resection will allow fluid to accumulate obligatorily without an indication for inserting a chest drain in such spaces.

In general, when assessing the indication for a chest drain for fluid removal, one must define whether a thoracentesis (single or multiple) has the same or even a better outcome then a chest drain for a determined time period.

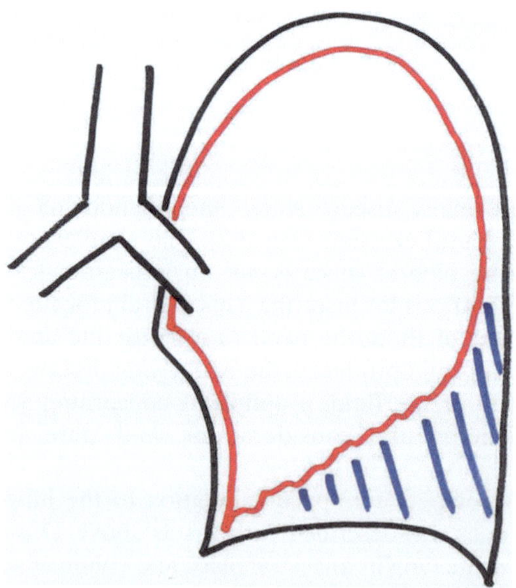

Figure 3.2 Pleural effusion: typical localisation dorsobasal

3.1.3   Redirecting of Fluid

The below named reasons could lead to an indication for draining fluid not extra-thoracic but instead into another anatomic compartment (i.e. intraabdominal) (Fig. 3.3). A potential benefit is that the fluid is not lost but instead remains in the body. Long term extra thoracic drainage of fluid has the potential to lead to complications which could include malnutrition.

3.1.4   Pressure Relief

The accumulation of gas, air, or fluid may, under distinct circumstances, lead to the development of significant intrathoracic pressure that is detrimental to the respiratory and/or the

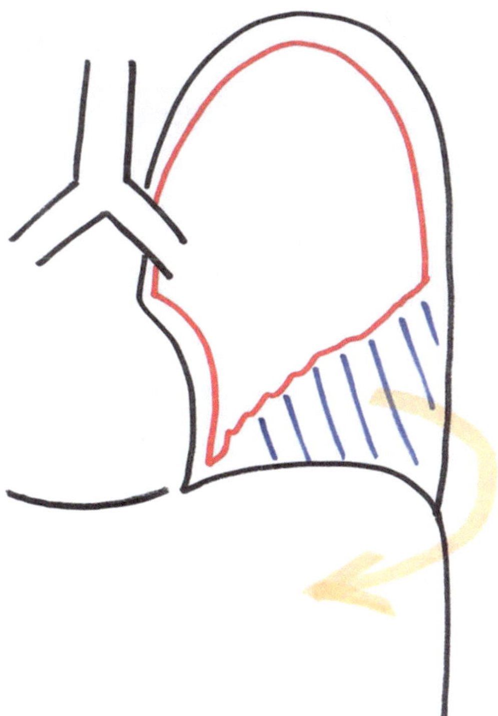

FIGURE 3.3 Thoraco-abdominal bypass

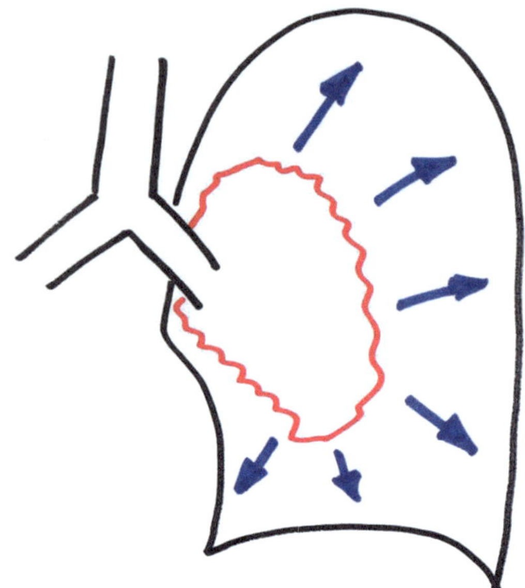

FIGURE 3.4 Unphysiological intrathoracic pressure

cardiac systems (Fig. 3.4). This may necessitate emergent chest drainage. Taking into consideration the probability of recurrence and underlying disease dynamics, the indication in this setting may be thoracentesis versus insertion a chest drain for immediate relief.

3.1.5   Expanding Passive Atelectasis

Competition of fluid or gas/air with lung volume leads to the development of atelectasis by compression of the lung parenchyma (Fig. 3.5). There is a reduction of the vital capacity and eventually dyspnea may occur. Another consideration for inserting a chest drain is if the pleural fluid is rich in protein, fibrin, hemorrhagic, or is even pure blood. This leads quite quickly to the development of a rind covering the surface of the lung, followed by compression and atelectasis, resulting in

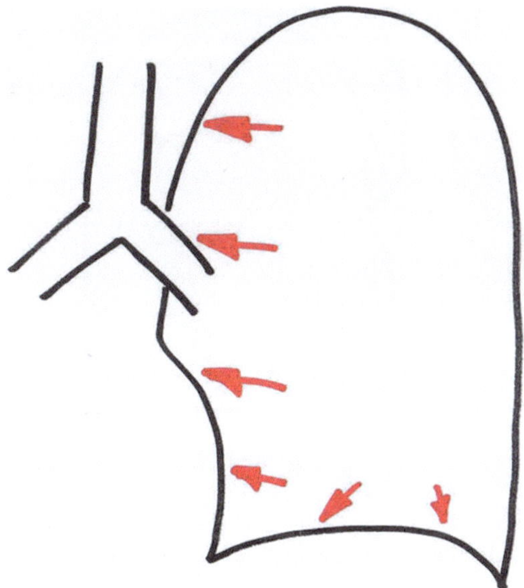

FIGURE 3.5 Expansion of atelectasis

a situation where even a sufficiently placed chest drain is no longer able to encourage lung reexpansion. Timing of chest drainage under these conditions is a very important issue as the success of the therapy is related to when the drain is placed during the clinical course.

3.1.6   Application of Drugs Via the Drain

Chest drains may not only be used for relief or evacuation of air/gas/fluid but also to act as a route to allow potentially therapeutic medications to be instilled into the chest cavity (Fig. 3.6). The probability of reaching the target area in the chest cavity and the anticipated success rate have to be taken into consideration when considering such a procedure. Whether the instruments used for this are able to fulfil the task is another question.

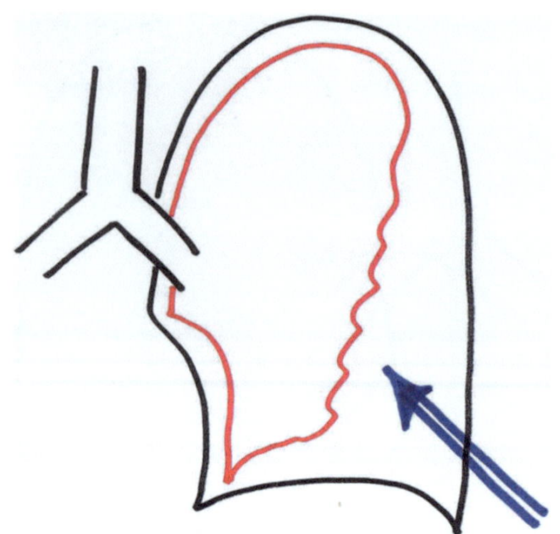

FIGURE 3.6 Instillation of medications into the pleural space

3.2   Drainage of Air/Gas

3.2.1   *Pneumothorax*

3.2.1.1   Primary Spontaneous Pneumothorax

Chest drain insertion for primary spontaneous pneumothorax (PSP) can address several potential therapeutic goals such as management of an emergency situation, monitoring of a broncopleural fistula, and potential treatment of an underlying disease. The first goal is to evacuate the air from the pleural space that may be a consequence of a leak in the lung parenchyma allowing air to accumulate. At the same time, this should facilitate the more or less collapsed lung tissue to reexpand (Fig. 3.7) followed by restoration and maintenance of subatmospheric pressure in the pleura space.

In the setting of lung collapse with significant positive pressure within the chest, a tension pneumothorax can arise necessitating an emergent chest drain. In primary or spontaneous pneumothorax, per definition, the pleura and lung

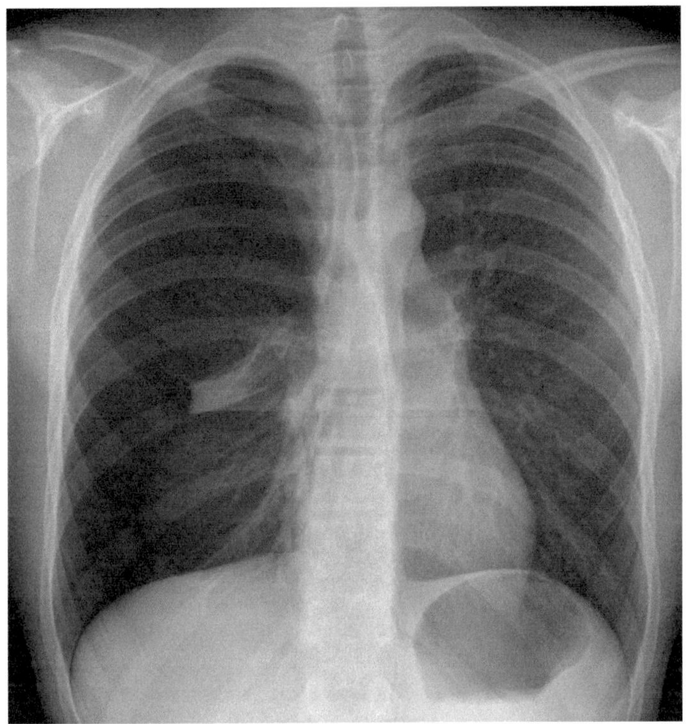

FIGURE 3.7 Primary spontaneous pneumothorax without tension

tissue are not diseased and therefore insertion of a chest drain can proceed in the usual fashion.

The necessity for chest drainage is in most cases given and depends on the quantitative occurrence of the pneumothorax and on the clinical symptoms (Klopp et al. 2007) [1].

The US-American (ACCP) an well as the British societies (BTS) offer guidelines for the treatment of primary spontaneous pneumothorax (Baumann et al. 2001; MacDuff et al. 2010), although both guidelines do not have the same results on all issues. One must recognize that there is only a small group of patients eligible for a purely conservative approach without thoracentesis or chest tube insertion (i.e. a "small" pneumothorax without any clinical symptoms). Even in this situation, the literature is not clear in its definition of what constitutes a "small" pneumothorax and differ concerning symptoms. The ACCP uses the distance from the apex of the lung to the upper end of the chest in its definition, whereas the BTS measures the distance from lung surface at the level of the hilum to the chest wall. In summary, only the "small" asymptomatic pneumothorax with less than 1 cm distance between lung and chest wall can be treated without procedural intervention.

In all other clinical settings the air should be evacuated. This can be done by thoracentsis with needle aspiration (Devanand et al. 2004) or by inserting a small bore catheter placed with a hollow-bore needle. Due to a low success rate this procedure is not recommended in infants (Soccorso et al. 2015). Needle aspiration is also not able to monitor any potential ongoing parenchymal leak. Small bore catheters are able to evacuate air (Vedam and Barnes 2003) but these catheters tend to clog quite fast because of fibrin so that ongoing safe function is not guaranteed. This is one of the reasons that frequently a 20 F catheter is therefore used.

If there is clinical concern for the presence of an on-going air leak, a large bore catheter (20–32 F) should be chosen. With these larger bore catheters, higher flow rates can be managed so that the occurrence of subcutaneous emphysema is less frequent. One must remember though that in an acute life threatening tension pneumothorax, simple needle aspiration can provide initial pressure relief as to allow the subsequent chest drain insertion to be done in a more controlled fashion.

The insertion of a chest drain for spontaneous pneumothorax should restore the physiological conditions in the pleural space. The chest tube remains for a defined period of time working as a monitoring tool and may possibly be the only therapeutic procedure needed. Exact rules for post procedural therapeutic course are not consistent (ACCP and BTS). In the end existing risk factors and other patient specific parameters must be taken into account when making an individualized therapeutic decision.

There are very few situations where a drain placement for primary spontaneous pneumothorax is not indicated.

3.2.1.2   Secondary Pneumothorax

There are numerous disease states that may cause a secondary pneumothorax (SPX). Pathological changes in the lung parenchyma such as what is seen in chronic obstructive pulmonary disease or interstitial lung disease (Ichinose 2015) are underlying factors. When a chest tube is indicated in the setting of a spontaneous pneumothorax, the clinician must be aware that therapy can be significantly complicated by severe changes in lung parenchyma (i.e. giant bullae) or abnormalities of the pleural space (i.e. pleural adhesions) Fig. 3.8.

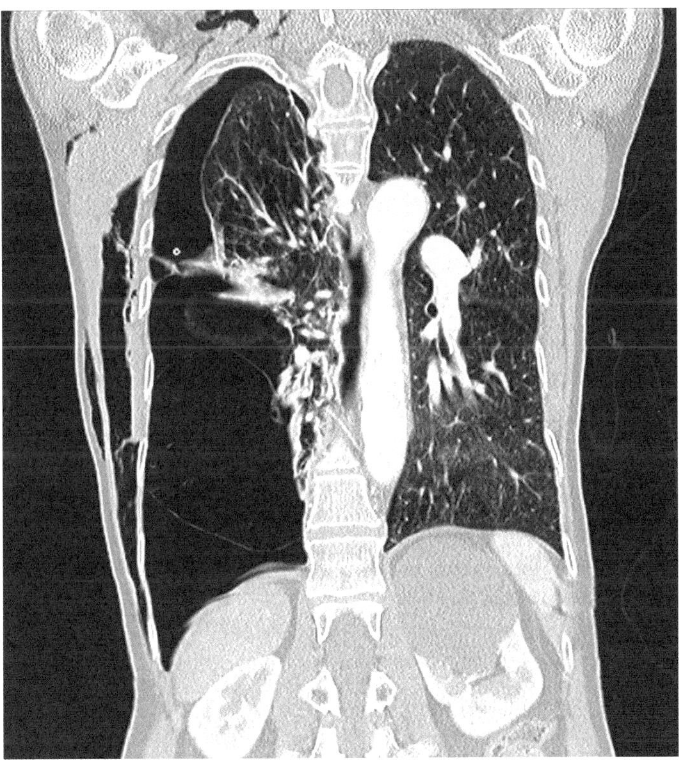

FIGURE 3.8 Pneumothorax and giant bulla

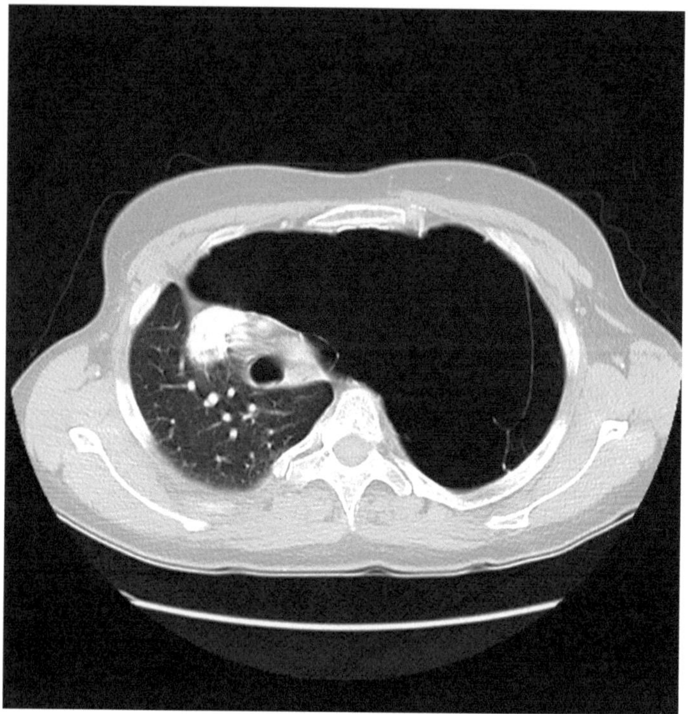

FIGURE 3.9 Simulated pneumothorax in case of giant bulla

In some cases parenchymal changes such as a giant bulla can be misinterpreted as a pneumothorax (Fig. 3.9). Such an abnormality is not an indication for chest tube insertion and iatrogenic complications can arise such as organ perforation.

Pneumothoraces in the setting of interstitial lung disease and cystic fibrosis are associated with high rates of complications and even mortality (Flume et al. 2010). Sufficient drainage has to be established quickly. Needle aspiration has been shown to be an inferior procedure in these patients.

In the case of a SPX there is almost always an indication to insert a chest drain as was described previously. If there is a significant risk of an air leak, a drain larger than 20 F is indicated in most cases. In the setting of an insufficiently drained pneumothorax (drain in the fissure, covered by lung tissue, on-going large air leak, etc.), the patient must be quickly reassessed for possible insertion of a second tube or if the previous tube should be replaced with a single new tube.

Patients with a secondary pneumothorax may have changes in the pleural cavity (postoperative, post inflammatory, etc.) which can cause difficulties during chest drain insertion. This may lead to complications and subsequent harm. Giant bullous emphysema must also be taken into consideration!

3.2.2   *Iatrogenic Pneumothorax*

The proportion of iatrogenic pneumothoraces in all patients suffering from a pneumothorax is quite high. The main indication for chest tube insertion is to drain air from the pleural space and restore physiological conditions. Some patients may be able to be closely observed without needle aspiration or having a chest tube insertion inserted for management of an iatrogenic pneumothorax.

The patients suffering from iatrogenic pneumothoraces are heterogeneous. There are essentially two groups of patients with these pneumothoraces and should be separately considered when deciding on chest drainage. The first group have pneumothoraces that are related to biopsies and line insertions (Despars et al. 1994). "Small" asymptomatic pneumothoraces may be observed and treated without further invasive action in this group. All other instances in this group should be treated by needle aspiration or with insertion of a small bore catheter. If there is a large air leak present, this is an indication for insertion a larger bore catheter.

The second group of patients incur iatrogenic pneumothoraces from barotrauma from mechanical ventilation or are ventilated at the time of the first appearance of the (iatrogenic) pneumothorax. In these situations the risk of getting a tension pneumothorax is very high and therefore chest drain insertion is indicated. A small bore catheter in these circumstances is correlated with low success rate, and therefore the use of large bore (>20 F) is recommended.

Every pneumothorax in patients requiring mechanical ventilation must be drained!

3.2.3   Traumatic Pneumothorax

Traumatic pneumothoraces are not always due to a penetrating injury. It is important to note that more than 30 % of traumatic pneumothoraces are not detectable on conventional x-ray but only are identified with a CT scan (Yadav et al. 2010). When this occurs it is referred to as an "occult pneumothorax".

In general a traumatic pneumothorax presents an indication for insertion a chest drain. If there is just a pneumothorax, in the absence of simultaneous hemothorax, and without significant injuries of the lung parenchyma, there is no valid statement as to which drain diameter is recommended. In the case of dysfunction of a smaller bore catheter in this setting, the placement of a large bore catheter should be performed quite quickly. In trauma patients on the ventilator, a large bore (>20 F) catheter is recommended as well.

Only in an occult pneumothorax or in selected cases of a very small pneumothorax, is there an indication for clinical observation with serial x-rays over chest drainage. This treatment strategy should only be applied to nonventilated patients (de Lesquen et al. 2015). When clinical symptoms of a tension pneumothorax are identified, immediate pressure relief by placement of a drain is required.

Whenever a traumatic pneumothorax has to be drained, monitoring of the patient must be guaranteed.

3.2.4   Subcutaneous Emphysema

Subcutaneous emphysema can present a special clinical situation when encountered during the course of treatment of the above mentioned situations. This can even occur during chest tube therapy. Subcutaneous emphysema occurs, in particular, after draining a pneumothorax in a patient who is mechanically ventilated. In the literature it was presumed that this is a complication due to chest tube therapy.

Two situations have to be taken into consideration regarding further therapy:

On one hand there is often a "mismatch" between the amount of air in the pleural space caused by a high volume broncopleural fistula or caused/accelerated by strong breathing excursions (i.e. coughing) and the maximal drainage capacity of the chest tube. In this case, it has to be decided whether the chosen diameter of the tube is too small, potentially necessitating the addition of a second (or third) chest drain, or if the current drain needs to be upsized.

These additional drains have to be positioned in an optimal way in order to reach the existing pleural air space or to target the specific area of the thoracic cavity under concern.

On the other hand subcutaneous emphysema may be caused by the fact that the chest tube is not optimally functioning due to tissue covering part/all of the drainage holes (Fig. 3.10). In this situation the placement of a new chest drain is indicated.

The reason for subcutaneous emphysema developing or persisting after drainage therapy must found and if necessary, adequate procedures to solve the problem have to be undertaken. A passive strategy might be dangerous!

3.3   Fluid Drainage

3.3.1   Parapneumonic Effusion and Empyema

The incidence of pleural infections is high and these are associated with significant morbidity and mortality. There are a number of medical strategies for diagnosis. The placement of a chest tube has the ability to obtain fluid for analysis and the potential for treatment. There are attempts to stratify this therapeutic plurality in guidelines (Davies et al. 2010).

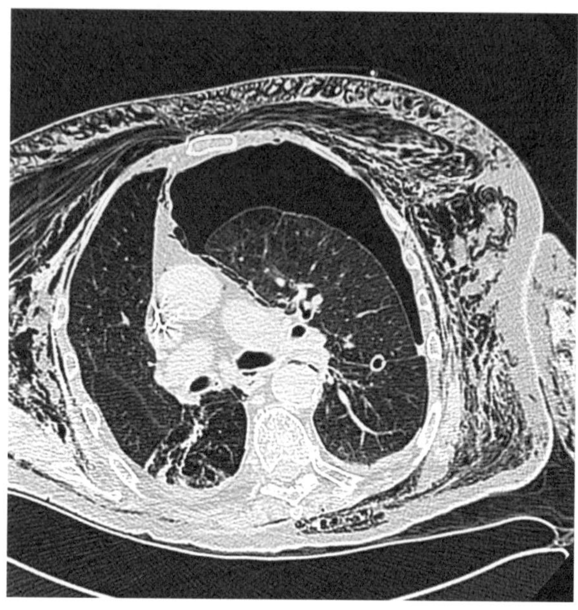

FIGURE 3.10 Subcutaneous emphysema caused by malfunction of the chest tube

It has to be emphasized that pleural infections are rarely diseases having a distinct status but instead are constantly changing in the morphology and consistency of the pleural fluid. This is important with regard to the indications for inserting a chest tube. Very often the fluid is not free floating in the chest cavity, and instead is loculated with multiple fluid filled compartments found. These compartments again are in different states of development representing the disease's dynamic changing nature (Fig. 3.11).

At the same time, the pleura is also undergoing change which has been observed to compromise lung function (visceral rind or constrained atelectasis). These findings on their own represent a disease process and appropriate therapeutic actions have to follow. These discussions show how difficult it is to develop guidelines for treatment, including chest tube therapy, of parapneumonic effusions and pleural empyemas.

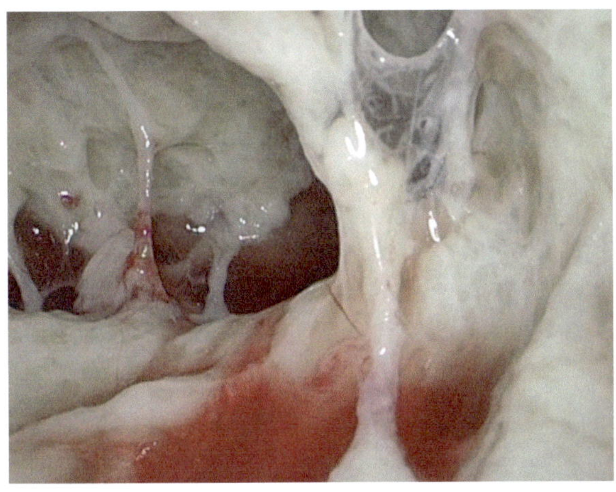

FIGURE 3.11 Fibro-purulent, partitioned empyema

Thoracentesis is indicated if a pleural effusion is a complication of pneumonia, if there is suspicion for infection, and if the effusion is freely floating within the chest cavity. Aspiration in this setting is for diagnostic purposes although complete evacuation of the fluid should be the aim due to pragmatic reasons. Quite often a single aspiration may represent a definitive therapy. Recurrence of a parapneumonic effusion occurs very often in a quite dynamic way (<24 h). In this setting a chest drain is indicated as a diagnostic tool and for monitoring the effusion and the disease respectively. Discussion is ongoing whether a small bore or a large bore tube should be used in this situation. Small bore catheters have a higher rate of failure in particular when used in patient's with a pleural empyema. An exchange for a large bore catheter may need to be quickly undertaken as morbidity and disease duration will be determined by the adequacy of the drainage. The instillation of enzymes may be considered during this stage of the disease as the quality of the effusion changes towards a more protein and fibrin rich morphology. The drainage system has to be adapted to accommodate this fluid change.

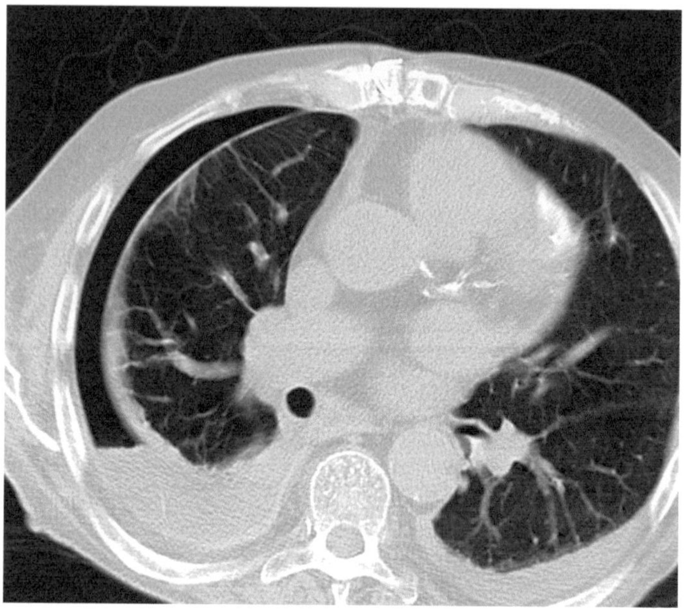

FIGURE 3.12 Visceral rind

A large bore tube is definitely indicated during the transition from a stage I (exudative) of pleural infection to a stage II (purulent) infection. Individualized protocols may necessitate more chest tubes or special "rinse" tubes. During this stage of the disease, it is quite common for chest tube treatment to fail as the there is development of a visceral rind. This leads to a situation where the lung is no longer able to fully expand even if the treatment of the pleural empyema is successful (Figs. 3.12 and 3.13).

In the presence of a pleural effusion caused by an inflammatory process, there are pleural changes at the surface of the lung and the diaphragm which have a pathologic impact. Successful therapy is dependent on the timing of the intervention!

Therapeutic strategies must take into account the heterogeneity of findings, the capability to define the correct stage of the disease, and the early dynamic changes that may

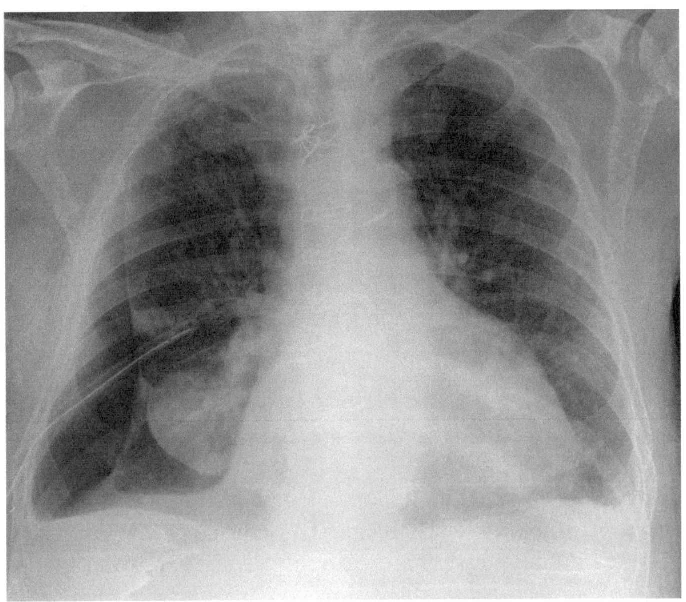

FIGURE 3.13 Captured lung

worsen the disease. These components play an important roll and need to be simultaneously approached with a stage adopted therapy to provide the patients with the best treatment. These requirements may be best satisfied by video assisted thoracoscopic surgery (Bilgin et al. 2006). Surgery allows for the exact positioning of a chest tube under direct view and, if necessary, also the stage adopted installation of a rinse system. When possible, drains should be placed in a way that allow for treatment of the entirety of the pleural disease. In a stage II pleura empyema, the indication for surgery becomes more evident but the patient must be assessed for risk of surgical intervention. In septic patients the increase in anesthetic and perioperative risk involving surgery may be too high. In this setting a chest tube may be indicated to attempt to detoxify now for surgery later on under improved conditions.

With stage III (organized) pleural infections, open decortication is indicated. If due to acute clinical considerations surgery is not suitable, chest drain therapy may be applied to attempt to halt progression of an abscess or even an empyema, while patient is stabilized empyema while the patient is stabilized.

When a pleural empyema involves pleural compartments (loculations) this may increase recurrence rates and therefore may indicate image guided placement of a drain (i.e. pigtail drain).

All drainage and therapeutic procedures for inflammatory pleural effusions must be monitored for their effectiveness shortly after the intervention.

3.3.2 *Malignant Pleural Effusion*

The treatment of a malignant pleural effusion may involve the insertion of a chest drain. The consideration for chest tube treatment must center around the fact that the malignant pleural effusion is a symptom of an underlying disease with an extremely poor prognosis (Ried and Hofmann 2013). Multiple diseases can cause this problem (Table 3.1).

Chest drain treatments in malignant pleural effusions seek to drain the effusion allowing reexpansion of the lung (to improve symptoms such as dypsnea) and allow for the installation of drugs for pleurodesis.

TABLE 3.1 Incidence of pleural carcinomatosis and malignant pleural effusion

Tumor entity (all Stages)	Patients with pleural carcinomatosis (%)	Primary tumor (Cytology) (%)	Estimated mean survival
Lung cancer	ca. 8–15	25–52	8-Jun
Breast cancer	ca. 2–12	27-Mar	Jun-48
Lymphoma	ca. 7	22-Dec	7-Jun
Other tumors	–	29–46	–

Ried and Hofmann (2013)

Pleural effusions can be massive leading to significant cardiopulmonary symptoms in patients with advanced malignant disease. Aspiration may be indicated in emergency situations to relieve symptoms. Repeated aspirations should only be done if life expectancy is less than four weeks because there is an increased infection risk with each additional instrumentation. When prognosis and survival are poor in end stage disease, the aim of drainage therapy is palliation of symptoms which can be effective with a small bore catheter (i.e. via Seldinger technique). Such a procedure should be performed early after the appearance of a malignant effusion as the risk of a restrictive visceral rind due to partly hemorrhagic effusions is high. In addition, one can determine if there will be the ability to achieve visceral and parietal pleura apposition. This information is crucial when deciding if someone would benefit from a pleurodesis.

If pleural fluid production is very high, evacuation of the effusion should be performed in a way that no more than 1500 ml/day are drained to prevent reexpansion edema (Fig. 3.14). The risk is particularly high if pulmonary lymphangiosis is present at the same time.

If a chest tube is inserted to evacuate an effusion and possibly be used for pleurodesis, a small bore tube may be justified if the drug to be instilled can be prepared as a solution (doxycycline, bleomycin, etc.). The most effective pleurodesis can be achieved by using talc. It is not possible to prepare talc in a solution but in a suspension. That is why after installation local accumulation is often observed, in particular in the recesses next to the diaphragm. Talc poudrage is more effective (Stefani et al. 2006) where talc is spread homogenously in the pleural cavity. This is another reason why a thoracoscopic surgical approach is more efficient because of direct placement of a tube, ability to biopsy for diagnosis, and talc poudrage can all be completed in one procedure. At the end of the surgery the chest tube stays in place and is then used as monitoring tool until the pleurodesis is effective and the effusion is stopped.

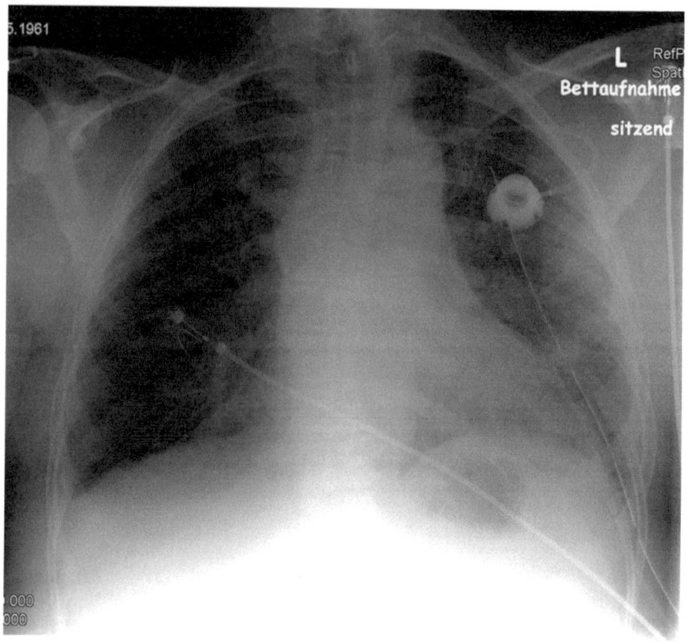

FIGURE 3.14 Early stage of reperfusion edema after draining of a large pleural effusion

If pleurodesis is unsuccessful, a clinically relevant recurrent effusion occurs, or if pleurodesis is no longer possible due to shrinkage of the lung, a permanent pleural catheter is indicated (PleurX® Drainage-System, CareFusion Germany, Kelberg, Germany). This system can stay in situ over the course of the disease without affecting the patient's hygiene or mobility. The permanent pleural catheter can clog due to fibrin but this can be solved with instillation of fibrinolytics. There is a 60 % chance of "spontaneous" pleurodesis which could allow for eventual ability to remove the drain.

When significant hemorrhagic effusions are encountered, tubes with an adequate diameter (20 F) should be used to avoid dysfunction (i.e. clogging). Relevant bleeding from pleural carcinomatosis would indicate the use of rinse tubes.

If pleurodesis is indicated for management of a malignant pleural effusion, this procedure should be done early on in the course of the disease. The therapeutic and/or palliative procedure has to be chosen according to the prognosis of the individual disease.

3.3.3   Benign Pleural Effusion

If clinical evaluation rules out the presence of a pleural effusion caused by the above mentioned etiologies (parapneumonic, malignant, or traumatic), a chest drain is indicated in the presence of a clinical relevant pleural effusion.

Aspiration of the pleural effusion is a key point in diagnosis. The literature has recommendations about pleural transudates and exudates and how to narrow the differential diagnosis (Hooper et al. 2010):

A transudate may be due to such causes as left heart insufficiency, a functional disorder of the liver, or a nephrotic syndrome. There are numerous other causes with some of them being very rare. There is an 85 % chance that the pleural effusion will disappear as the underlying disease is treated successfully and therefore chest drainage is rarely indicated. Very few cases need pleurodesis due to recurrence. A chest tube is then used as a monitoring tool to observe the circadian dynamics of the effusions production. If pleurodesis is needed, a chest drain system has to be chosen which optimizes this method and the agent to be used.

In the presence of an exudative effusion, the most common etiologies are malignant, parapneumonic, or related to a specific pleural disease. The indication for drainage is already discussed above. When discussing diagnostic and therapeutic options, pleuritis, benign pleural disease, and mesothelioma must be taken into consideration. In both settings there may be a need for pleural biopsy. If biopsy and drainage is needed, this can efficiency be completed during a thoracoscopic procedure whereby a chest tube is left to monitor and continue to drain any fluid. The early development of fluid filled compartments (loculations) is common with pleural exudates. This can cause parts of the lung to shrink due to atelectasis. Incidental pleural aspirations (i.e. with underlying diseases such as from rheumatoid disease) should be avoided in favor of a temporary treatment with a chest tube. Small bore tubes are usually sufficient in this case.

Pleural effusions that are not caused by trauma, inflammation, or malignancy should be meticulously analyzed before any drainage procedure is done.

3.3.3.1   Pleural Effusion After Cardiac Surgery

Pleural effusions following cardiac surgery, most often after bypass surgery, represent a special entity of benign exudative pleural effusions. It is not appropriate to assume a common etiology. The etiologies for such an effusion include temporary cardiac insufficiency, a post operative hemothorax, postpericardiotomy syndrome, and chylothorax after preparation of the internal mammary artery. A conservative trial of treatment is justified in most cases (Light et al. 2002). Failure of treatment has to be noticed early and then chest drain therapy is indicated. When chest tube drainage no longer sufficiency drains the effusion, as with parapneumonic effusions, thoracoscopic intervention should be undertaken. The main goal is the prevention and/or removal of any consolidated or organized pleural formations.

Pleural effusions after cardiac surgery that do not decrease under sufficient conservative treatment must be drained in a reasonable timeframe.

3.3.4   Chylothorax

The spectrum of diseases that cause a chylous or pseudochorus effusion is broad, reaching from benign entities to malignancy, but the indication for initial drainage is uniform. Chest tube placement also allows for circadian monitoring of the effusions production (Fig. 3.15).

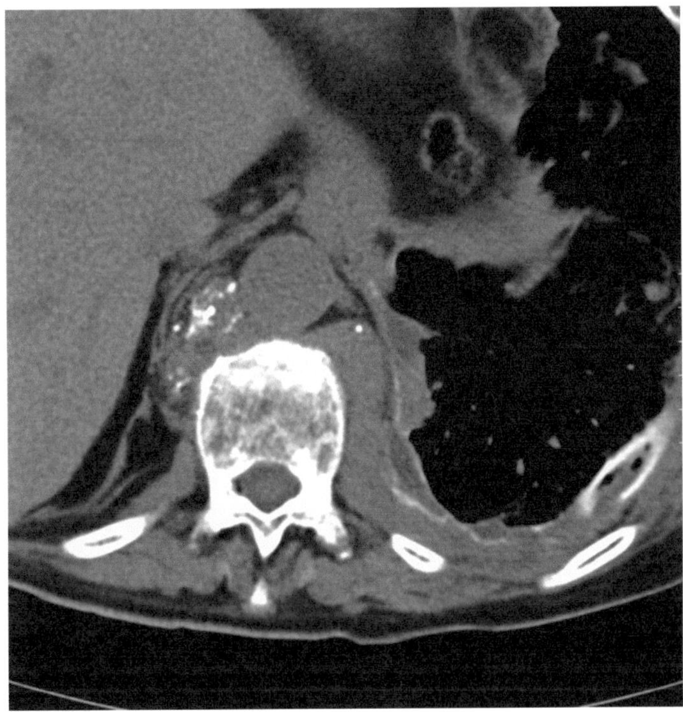

FIGURE 3.15 Lymphography showing contrast agent leakage to the left chest cavity directly drained by the chest tube.

There are a variety of treatment modalities to specifically address the underlying disease state: change in diet, drug therapy, interventional radiology procedures, and surgery (Bender et al. 2016). For treatment, chest drainage is indicated once again as a monitoring tool of fluid production and for documenting the success of the specific treatment. The distinct configuration of the chest tube in this situation is not clear in the literature. It can be assumed that small bore aspiration catheters as well as chest tubes with larger diameters can be used for these patients.

When the therapeutic algorithm includes drug pleurodesis or pleurectomy, a large bore tube (>20 F) should be used.

The risk of a drain induced infection is low and thus there is no indication for a rinse tube.

Chylous effusion should always be drained initially.

3.3.5 *Hemothorax*

Most hemothoraces develop due to a chest trauma. Other etiologies that can cause a hemothorax include malignant diseases of the pleura and spontaneous bleeding under systemic anticoagulation (Fig. 3.16).

Drainage of a hemothorax is indicated irrespective of the underlying etiology. Due to the consistency of hemothoraces, a

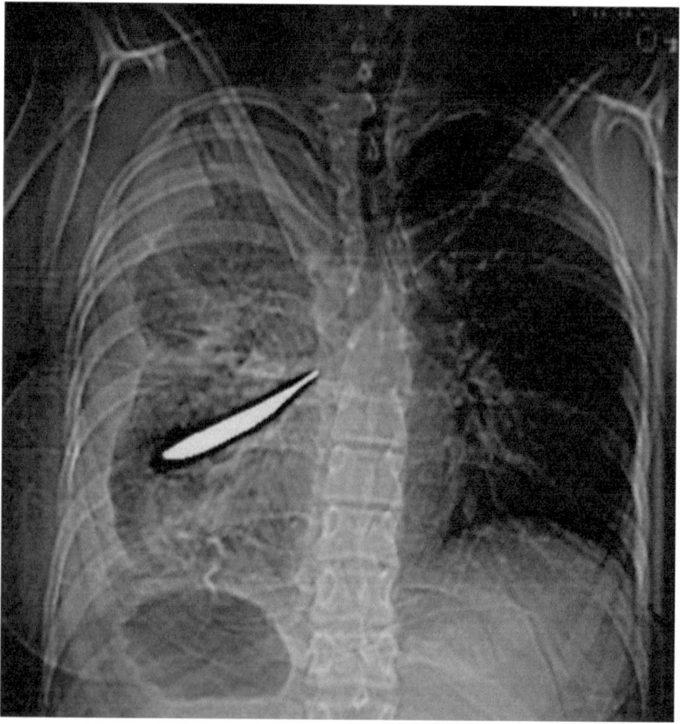

FIGURE 3.16 Hemothorax caused by stab wound

TABLE 3.2 Objective when draining a hemothorax

Complete evacuation of blood from the pleural space

Monitoring of the amount of blood and the activity of bleeding

Improved hemostasis due to apposition of the pleural sheets

Avoiding consecutive problems such as chronic atelectasis or pleural empyema

large bore catheter (>24 F) should be placed initially. Drainage is emphasized by the following objectives (Table 3.2):

A traumatic hemothorax is frequently present with a concurrent pneumothorax and therefore called a hemopneumothorax. The indication for drainage has been discussed previously (see above). More than one chest drain may need to be placed in order to obtain the therapeutic objectives.

Hemothorax treated with chest drainage alone has a high rate of treatment failure but the tube can be used as an important initial monitoring tool. The adequate function of the chest drain system must be ensured to avoid future complications such as chronic atelectasis. If there is any doubt about the efficiency of the chest drain system, an additional chest drain should be placed. If additional tubes are under consideration there also should be a discussion for thoracoscopic exploration of the chest. It cannot be expected that prolonged insufficient hemothorax drainage will improve over the time delivering good results.

Every hemothorax should be drained early. The chosen drainage system has to be adequate as short term control dictates the success of the therapy.

3.4   Redirection of a Pleural Effusion

There are a few special situations where drainage systems can be used to redirect a pleural effusion.

In these instances, exceptional steps are taken when a previous therapeutic algorithm is partially or completely unsuccessful. This may occur in the treatment of high volume chylous effusions and those pleural effusions due to massive ascites. Depending on the composition of the fluid, a patient's clinical status may worsen when significant proteins are lost and is therefore a reason to redirect the fluid.

In these cases, the fluid will be redirected to another compartment of the body (i.e. intraabdominal) to aid in reabsorption into the intravascular space to reduce the loss of proteins. The available system for this is the Denver®-Shunt (Denver®-Shunt, CareFusion Germany, Kelberg, Germany). Fluid can be redirected pleuro-peritoneal, pleuro-venous, or peritoneal-venous. When considering such a procedure, the indication for use, the pathophysiology of the underlying disease, any potential complications, and a risk-benefit calculation must be discussed (Perera et al. 2011). After implantation of a Denver®-Shunt the pleural cavity should be drained using it as long as the shunt works without complications.

The redirection of a pleural effusion to another body cavity is a individualized procedure that must be precisely indicated.

3.5   Postoperative Drainage

Postoperative drainage of the chest cavity is indicated in all procedures in which there is a possibility of the perioperative accumulation of air, serous fluids or blood in the chest cavity. This applies to many surgical procedures in thoracic surgery, as well as cardiac surgery, esophageal surgery, vascular surgery, neurosurgery, and orthopedic surgery.

The basic principle is to evacuate any air and/or fluid from the pleural space and the mediastinum. The drainage system chosen needs to fulfil these requirements (Table 3.3):

To fulfill these requirements, different configurations are favored according to individual preferences. Often drainage consisting of at least two tubes will be used in order to achieve an "air-drain" ventroapical and a "fluid-drain" dorsobasal or paravertebral approach (Fig. 3.17).

TABLE 3.3 Requirements of postoperative drainage of the chest cavity

Target orientated drainage: Sufficient drainage of the surgical site

Strategic localization of the drain: Appropriate to drain air sufficiently, if necessary with a high flow

Strategic localization of the drain: Appropriate to drain fluid sufficiently, if necessary anticipating pleural compartments developing later

Diameter of the chest tube: Appropriate to drain blood clots and fibrin (>24 F)

Optional: Possibility to rinse via special catheters

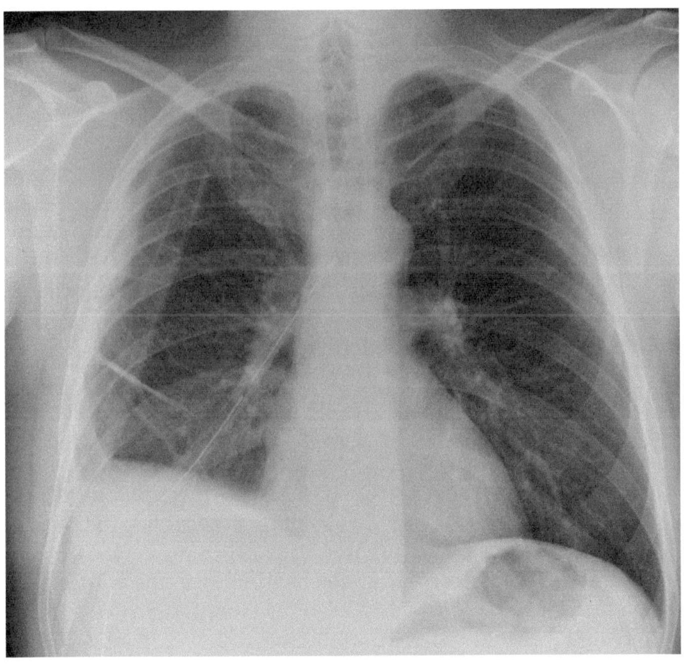

FIGURE 3.17 Typical postoperative drainage after lung resection with two drains

When a surgical site is contaminated or for surgery of septic diseases, special "rinse catheters" are indicated to guarantee sufficient cleaning of the surgical site or existing compartments in the postoperative period.

Postoperative pleural drainage should be based on standards that are defined by the individual center.

Literature

1. Klopp M, Dienemann H, Hoffmann H. Treatment of Pneumothorax. Chirurg. 2007;78(7):655–668.
2. Baumann M, Strange C, Heffner J et al. Management of Spontaneous Pneumothorax. An American Colllege of Chest Physicians Delphi Consensus Statement. Chest. 2001;119:590–602.
3. MacDuff A, Arnold A, Harvey J. on behalf of the BTS Pleural Disease Guideline Group. Management of spontaneous pneumothorax: British Thoracic Society pleural disease guideline Thorax. 2010;65(Suppl 2):ii18eii31.
4. Devanand A, Koh MS, Ong TH et al. Simple aspiration versus chest-tube insertion in the management of primary spontaneous pneumothorax: a systematic review. Respir Med. 2004;98(7):579–90.
5. Soccorso G, Anbarasan R, Singh M et al. Management of large primary spontaneous pneumothorax in children: radiological guidance, surgical intervention and proposed guideline. Pediatr Surg Int. 2015;31(12):1139–44.
6. Vedam H, Barnes DJ. Comparison of large- and small-bore intercostal catheters in the management of spontaneous pneumothorax. Int Med J. 2003;33:495e9.
7. Ichinose J, Nagayama K, Hino H. Results of surgical treatment for secondary spontaneous pneumothorax according to underlying diseases. Eur J Cardiothorac Surg. 2015;8:pij: ezv256.
8. Yarmus L, Feller-Kopman D. Pneumothorax in the crititcally ill patient. Chest. 2012;141(4): 1098–1105.
9. Flume PA, Mogayzel Jr PJ, Robinson KA et al. Cystic fibrosis pulmonary guidelines: pulmonary complications: hemoptysis and pneumothorax. Am J Respir Crit Care Med. 2010;182:298–306.

10. Despars JA, Sassoon CSH, Light RW. Significance of iatrogenic pneumothoraces. Chest. 1994;105:1147–50.
11. Yadav K, Jalili M, Zehtabchi S. Management of traumatic occult pneumothorax. Resuscitation. 2010;81(9): 1063–8.
12. de Lesquen H, Avro JP, Gust L et al. Surgical management for the first 48 h following blunt chest trauma: state of the art (excluding vascular injuries). Interact CardioVasc Thorac Surg. 2015;20:399–408.
13. Davies HE, Davies R, Davies C. On behalf of the BTS Pleural Disease Guideline Group. BTS-Guideline: Management of pleural infection in adults. Thorax. 2010; 65(Suppl 2): ii41–ii53
14. Ried M, Hofmann HS. Dtsch Arztebl Int. 2013;110(18):313–8.
15. Stefani A, Natali P, Casali C et al. Talc poudrage versus talc slurry in the treatment of malignant pleural effusion. A prospective comparative study. Eur J Cardiothorac Surg. 2006;30(6):827–32.
16. Hooper C, Lee G, Maskell N. On behalf of the BTS Pleural Guideline Group. BTS-Guideline: Investigation of a unilateral pleura effusion in adults. Thorax. 2010;65:ii4–ii17.
17. Light R, Rogers J, Moyers J et al. Prevalence and clinical course of pleural effusion at 30 days after coronary artery and cardiac surgery. Am J Respir Crit Care Med. 2002;166:1567–71.
18. Bender B, Murthy V, Chamberlain RS. The changing management of chylothorax in the modern era. Eur J Cardiothoracic Surg. 2016;49(1):18–24.
19. Perera E, Bhatt S, Dogra VS. Complications of denver shunt. J Clin Imaging Sci. 2011;1:6.

Chapter 4
Different Kinds of Drains (–Catheters)

Erich Hecker

4.1 Introduction

There are many ways to categorize thoracic/pleural drains and catheters. These instruments can be grouped according to their indication (pneumothorax, hemothorax, pleural empyema, post-operative), the consistency of the fluid that can be drained (exudate, transudate, pus, blood, chylus), for drainage of air, the way of drain is placed (open-surgically, by intervention (Seldinger-technique)), the internal parts of the chest drain for guiding the tube (trocar, blunt stab, peaked stab, sharpened stab), the material (polyvinyl chloride (PVC), polyethylene (PE), silicone, free of latex or latex containing), the evacuation system (water seal, Heimlich-valve), industrially manufactured "all-in-one-systems"), the physical principles of suction generation (passive, Heber-principle), the allocation of suction (wall suction: negative pressure/positive pressure, electric allocation or mobile,

E. Hecker
Klinik für Thoraxchirurgie, Ev. Krankenhausgemeinschaft Herne,
Castrop-Rauxel gGmbH, Hordeler Straße 7-9, 44651 Herne,
Germany
e-mail: e.hecker@evk-herne.de

© Springer International Publishing Switzerland 2017
T. Kiefer (ed.), *Chest Drains in Daily Clinical Practice*,
DOI 10.1007/978-3-319-32339-8_4

battery-driven), as well as according to the so called "digital" combined pump-/suction system (Atmos, Medela).

The fact that there is not a perfect drain fulfilling all possible requirements or a drainage system that can satisfy all possible demands is reflected in the variety of commercially available chest tubes and drainage systems. The relevant, clinically important aspects concerning the indication of insertion (Chap. 3), technique of insertion (Chap. 6), possible complications (Chap. 7), and drain management (Chaps. 5, 8, 9, and 10) are described there.

This chapter will focus on the principle of the drain construction as all of the principles involved in their operation derive from it.

4.2   Materials

Polyvinyl chloride (PVC), polyethylene (PE), and silicone are the materials of which commercial available drains are made.

Polyvinyl chloride (PVC) is produced by polymerization of acetylene and hydrogen chloride. Soft-PVC is used for medical indications: contains 30 % softeners and should only be used for a short time as these toxic softeners may be freed and are prone to protein debris clogging. PVC-drains need a thickness of more than 2 mm to achieve stability concerning their shape.

Polyethylene (PE) is produced by chain polymerization from ethane. The corresponding catheters can be produced with very thin walls offering a good ratio of inner and outer diameter. Typical examples are redon- and pigtail-drains.

Silicone is a substance with chemical bonds that are between inorganic and organic, in particular between silicates and organic polymers. They could be considered hybrids with a unique spectrum of features unreached by any other synthetic material. The addition of Si-H-groups to silicone-bounded vinyl groups integrated in the ends of the polymeric chains and with the help of the so-called Liquid-Rubber-Technique, this material has an extremely low viscosity. This allows it to be pressed into shapes with high elasticity and stability. Silicone is free of softeners and organic additives resulting in a high tolerance in tissue.

Latex is produced from the milky juice of the rubber tree (Hevea brasiliensis). This fluid is mainly used for the production of rubber by vulcanization. Elastic polymers that are polymerized on isoprene as monomers, polymerized to cis-1,4 polyisoprene are named "caoutchouc". This rubber may cause allergies with a prevalence of 3–20 % due to proteins which are detectable in very low concentrations.

Siliconized Latex Drains These drains are moistened with silicone and therefore are less allergenic. Siliconized latex can be used as long-term drain.

4.3   Drains Shapes and Sizes

Most chest drains (silicone) have a diameter spanning from 14 F to 32 F which are available in different shapes (straight, curved). The number of holes for evacuation of air and/or fluid differs depending on the manufacturer from 2 to 20 at the side or at the tip of the drain. All have a radiopaque stripe incorporated in the tube. The drains are tissue conserving, have a high stability towards suction (>50 mbar), and are suitable as long term drains (>14 days) (Figs. 4.1 and 4.2).

Some companies do offer silicone-drains with a stab (trocar) inside. These trocars are designed for optimal guidance and positioning of the chest tube. The trocars can end bluntly in the tube with an integrated plastic cap to prevent organ injuries shields the tip. Other suppliers offer drains with trocars having round or even sharpened tips to facilitate the penetration of the tissue. The hazards of these drains are discussed in detail in Chap. 7 (Figs. 4.3, 4.4, 4.5, and 4.6).

Rinse-Suction Drains have a large bore channel for suction and evacuation of air/fluid and a small bore channel normally used for installation of rinsing fluid (Fig. 4.7).

Capillary drains or Jackson-Pratt drains have multiple small channels or holes that lead to an increase surface area

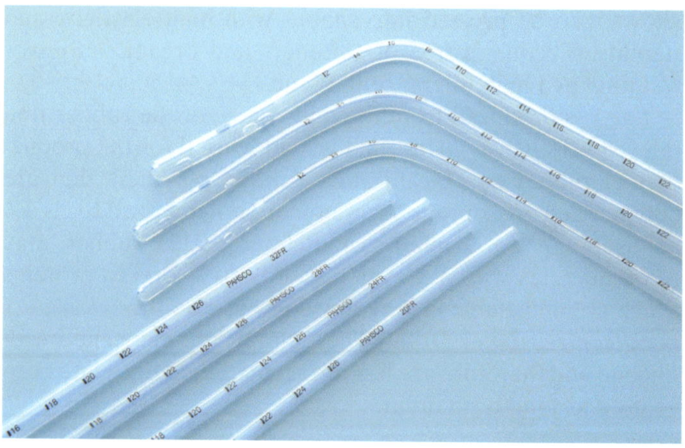

FIGURE 4.1 Chest tubes – straight and curved (Pacific Hospital Supply Co. Ltd, Fort Bend, Texas, USA)

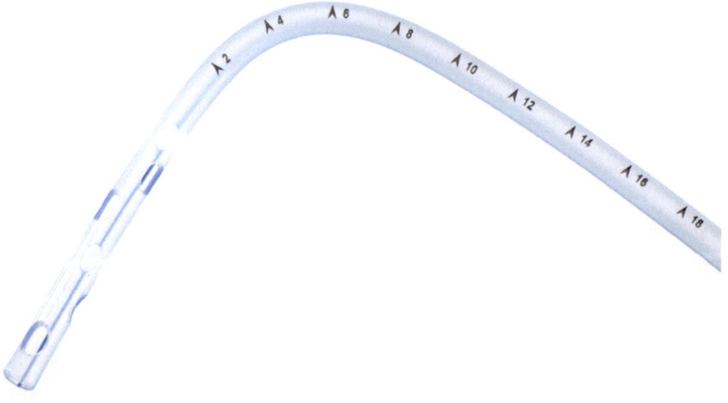

FIGURE 4.2 Curved chest tube with side holes (Free Life Medical GmbH, Aachen, Germany)

resulting in an increased diameter. At the same time the principle of capillary perforation is supposed to avoid clogging of the drain (Fig. 4.8).

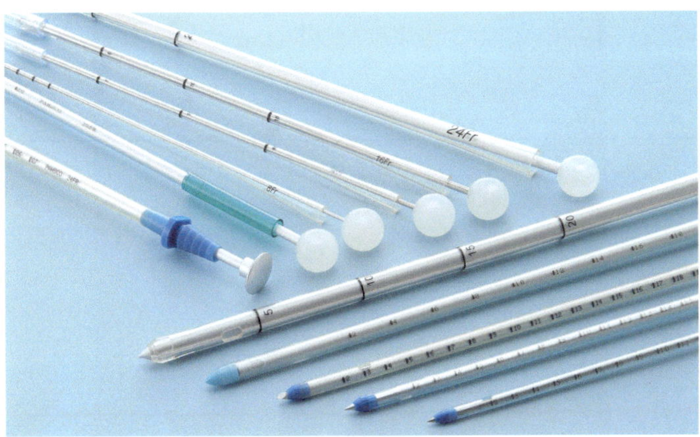

FIGURE 4.3 Chest tubes with Trocar (Pacific Hospital Supply Co. Ltd, Fort Bend, Texas, USA)

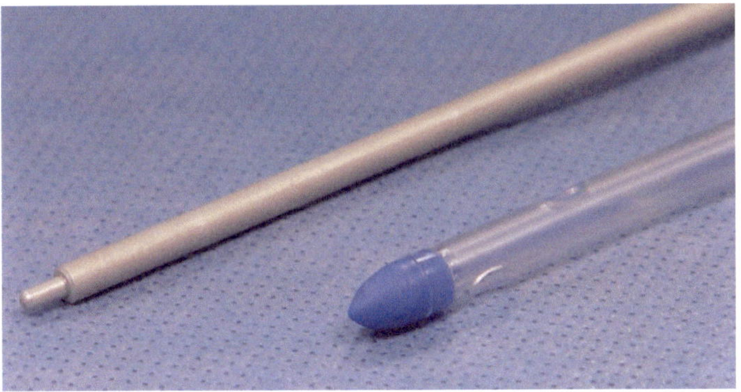

FIGURE 4.4 Trocar inside with protective cap (Schwandner G & G Klinikprodukte OG, St. Martin in Traun, Austria)

Aspiration drains are designed to evacuate air and fluid from the pleural space in an acute situation. Therefore the drains may be thin walled and are removed immediately after use. A Luer-Lock-connector is typically added to connect syringes or a evacuation bag. These catheters are made of silicone-polyethylene mixtures and should be removed at

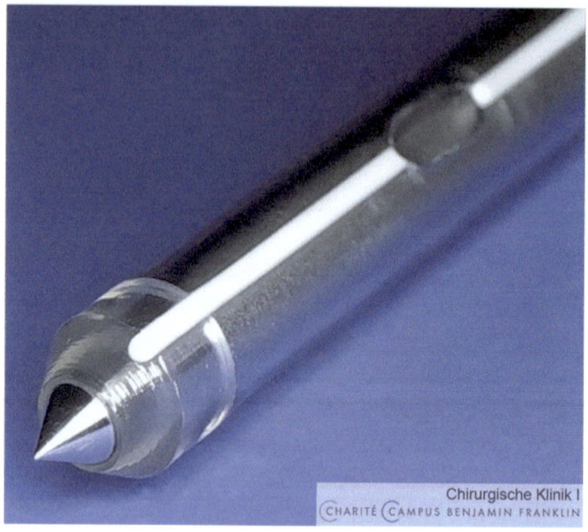

FIGURE 4.5 Chest tube with a sharpened Trocar (Supra Healthcare, Cape Town, Montague Gardens, South Africa)

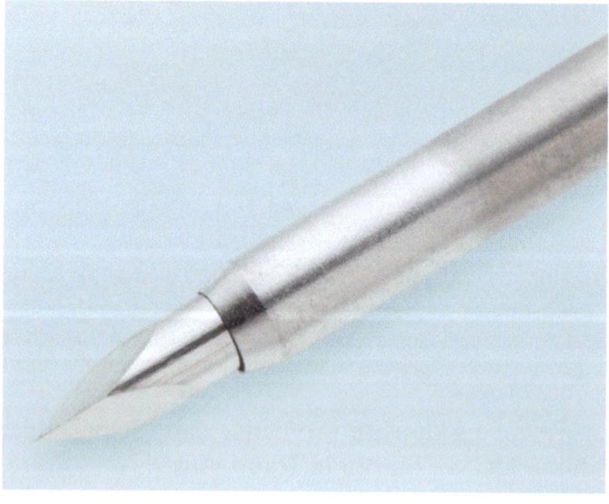

FIGURE 4.6 Chest tube with a sharpened Trocar (Somatex® Medical Technologies GmbH, Teltow, Germany)

least three days after initial use. Commercial available drains normally contain an application set (Redax SpA, Sede legale, Poggio Rusco, Italy) (Figs. 4.9 and 4.10).

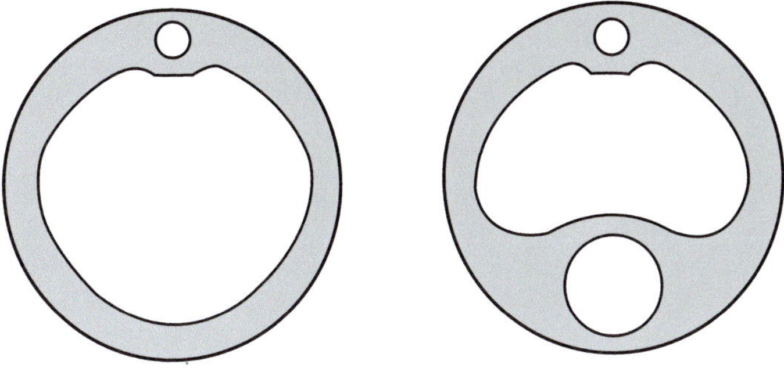

FIGURE 4.7 Rinse-Suction-Drain (single/double)

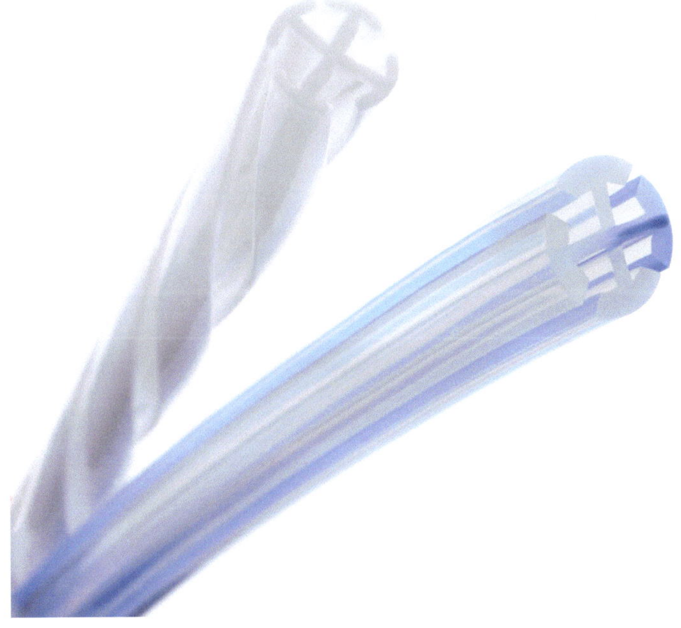

FIGURE 4.8 Jackson-Pratt drain

Pigtail-catheters are mainly used during CT or ultrasound guided interventions: The guide-wire or a trocar is placed in

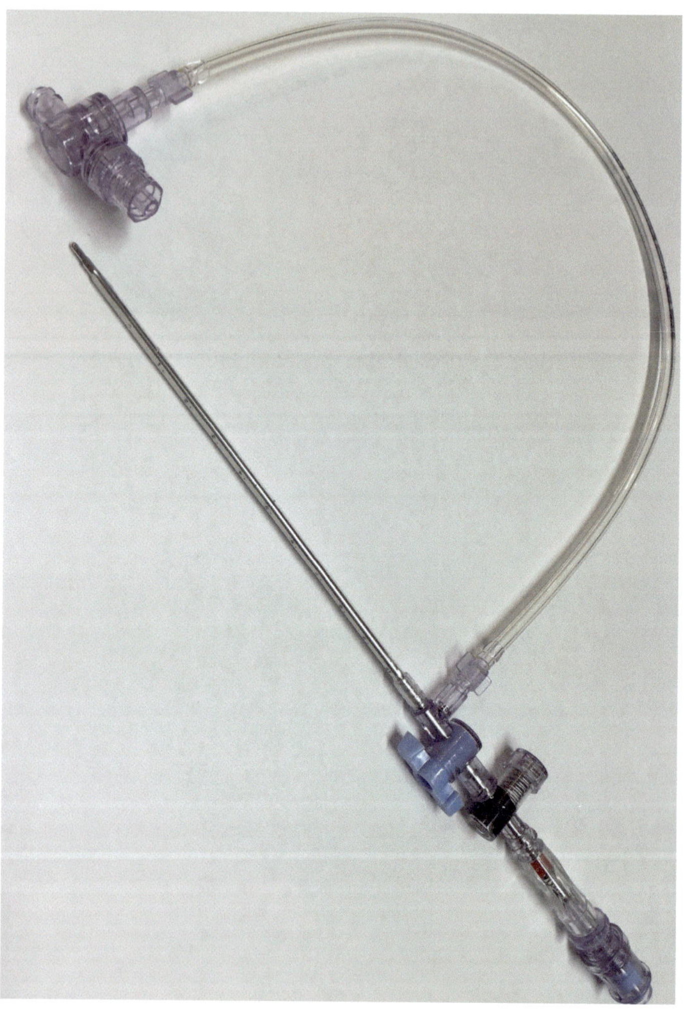

FIGURE 4.9 Aspiration drain without catheter

the target area followed by the definitive catheter which is guided by the wire or the cannula. The ability of the end of the catheter to corkscrew is created during the manufacturing process and gave the product its name ("pig tail"). This

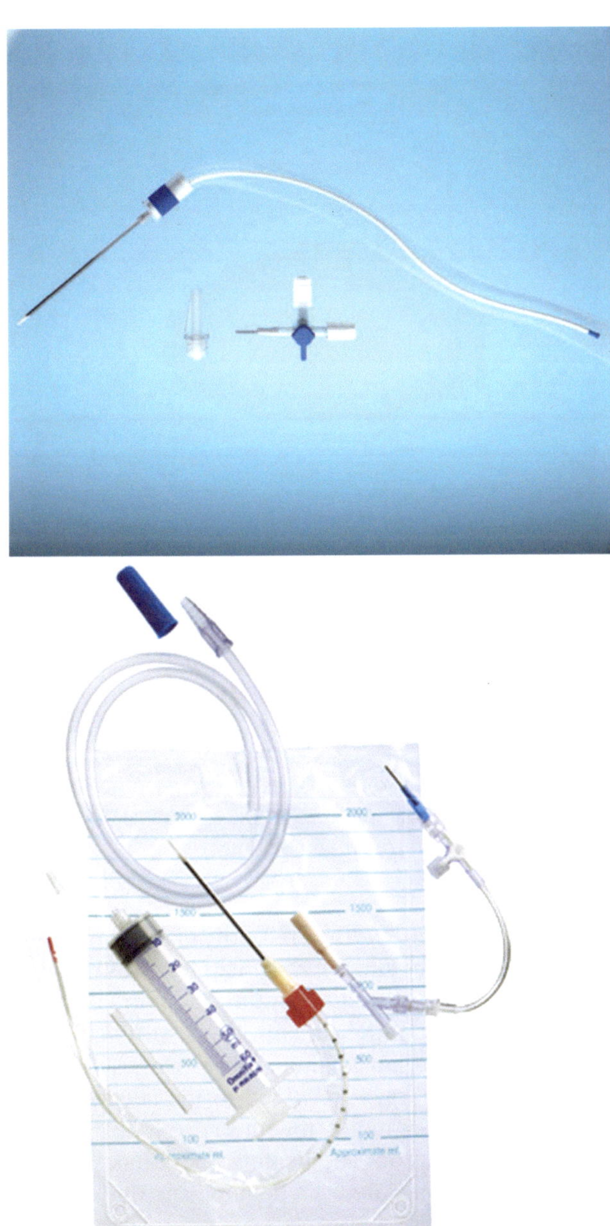

FIGURE 4.10 Aspiration drain with catheter and application set

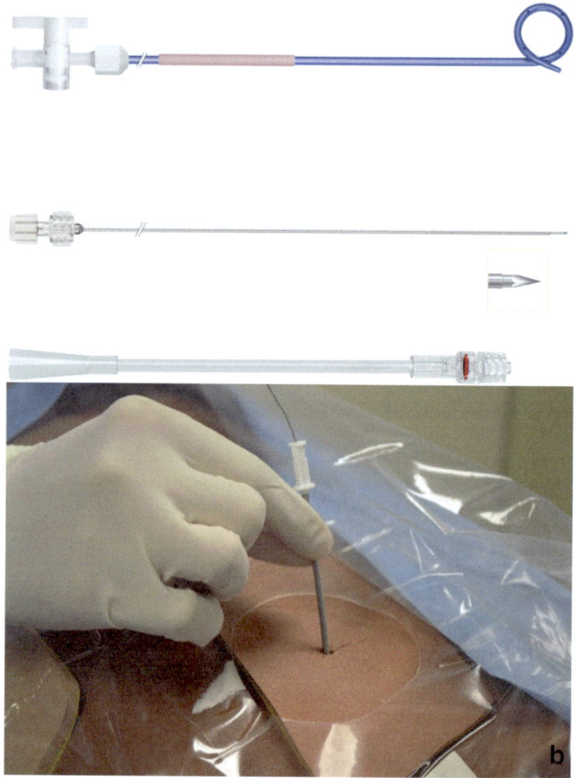

FIGURE 4.11 Pigtail with trocar and Seldinger-wire

configuration minimizes the risk of dislocation in situ (B. PraxiMed Vertriebs GmbH, Zwönitz, Germany) (Fig. 4.11).

A Redon-drain is a suction drain that normally is used after major surgery and left in situ. It is a stiff-walled drain made of polyethylene, having numerous perforations at its tip and a bottle with a "vacuum". Due to the suction applied, wound surfaces are brought together resulting in a faster development of adhesions and healing. Secretions (blood and serous fluid) are evacuated. Depending on the amount of

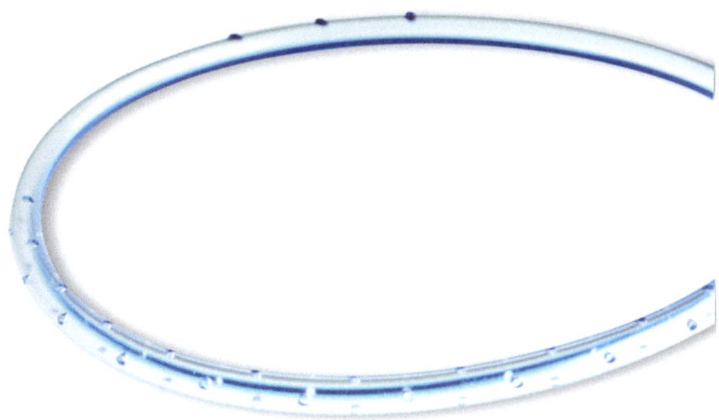

FIGURE 4.12 Redon drain

fluid produced, the drain is left in place for 48–72 h (A. Optimed Medizinische Instrumente GmbH, Ettlingen, Germany) (Fig. 4.12).

When permanent drain systems are needed, silicone tubes are chosen. With the help of a guide jacket and a subcutaneous tunnel, the drain is placed in the pleural space to allow for a permanent suction drain. The tube that resides in the subcutaneous tissue is reinforced with a polyester coating provoking an antibacterial inflammation followed by an incorporation of the tube into the tissue. Evacuation is done using gravity or by pre-fabricated suction bottles with a negative pressure according to the supplier (e.g. PleurX) of 50–200 mbar (Péters Surgical, Bobigny Cedex, France) (Fig. 4.13).

4.3.1   Filters

Commercial suppliers offer different filters for use with their chest drains. The benefit of these filters has not been shown in scientific studies. The main problems are that changes in fluid capacity are neither visible nor measurable, especially as the filter becomes wet or clogged. In such situations, the companies with an integrated system for suction and rinsing have

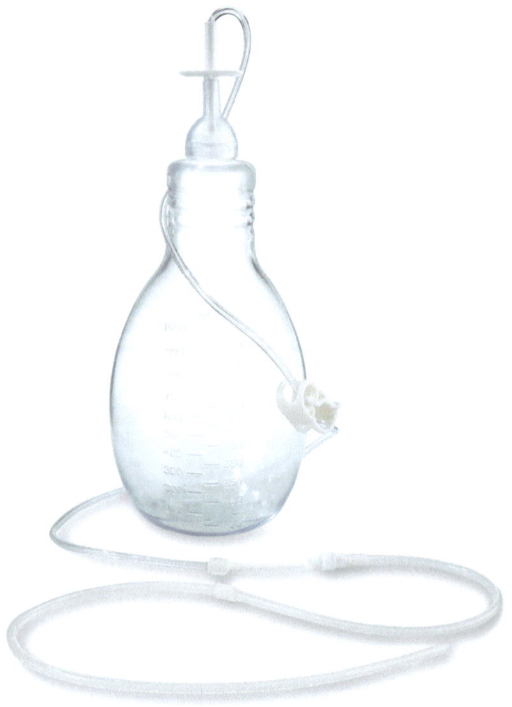

FIGURE 4.13 Permanent drain system

a significant advantage (Medela/Atmos) (MedCare, Boca Raton, USA) (Fig. 4.14).

The goal to evacuate air and/or fluid from the chest cavity can be achieved by any of the above listed drains. The selection of the proper drain is determined by the goal of therapy and by personal experience. When deciding on a "suction" or "no-suction" treatment approach, one must remember these patients need to be observed very carefully (P. J. Dahlhausen & Co. GmbH, Köln, Germany).

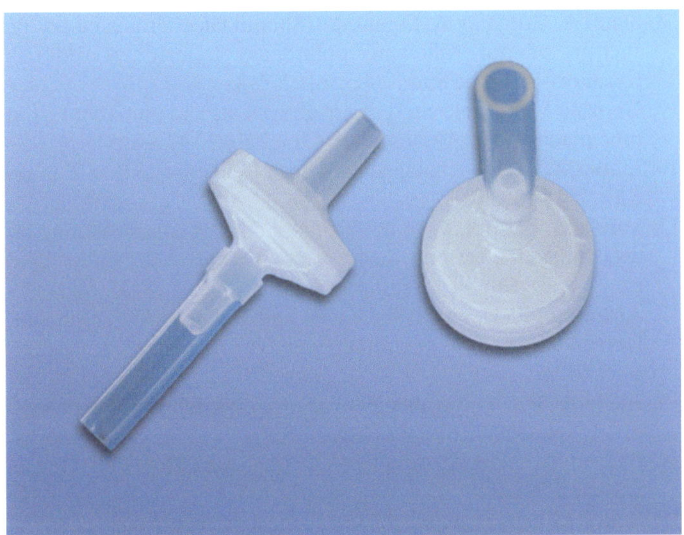

FIGURE 4.14 Filter

Literature

1. Kuhajda I, Zarogoulidis K, Kougioumtzi I, et al. Tube thoracostomy; chest tube implantation and follow up. J Thorac Dis. 2014;6 Suppl 4:470–9.
2. Daly RC, Mucha P, Pairolero PC, Farnell MB. The risk of percutaneous chest tube thoracostomy for blunt thoracic trauma. Ann Emerg Med. 1985;14(9):865–70.
3. Fishman NH. Thoracic drainage: a manual of procedures. Chicago: Year Book Medical Publishers; 1983.
4. Monaghan SF, Swan KG. Tube thoracostomy: the struggle to the "standard of care". Ann Thorac Surg. 2008;86(6):2019–22.
5. Gambazzi F, Schirren J. Thoracic drainage. What is evidence based? Chirurg. 2003;74(2):99–107.
6. Owen S, Gould D. Underwater seal chest drains: the patient's experience. J Clin Nurs. 1997;6(3):215–25.
7. Symbas PN. Chest drainage tubes. Surg Clin North Am. 1989;69(1):41–6.

8. Sanni A, Critchley A, Dunning J. Should chest drains be put on suction or not following pulmonary lobectomy? Interact Cardiovasc Thorac Surg. 2006;5(3):275–8.
9. Gonzalo V. Portable chest drainage systems and outpatient chest tube management. Thorac Surg Clin. 2010;20:421–6.
10. Linder A. Drainagemanagement nach Lungenresektion. Zentrbl Chir. 2014;139:50–8.
11. Varela G. Postoperative chest tube management: measuring air leak using an electronic device decreases variability in the clinical practice. Eur J Cardiothoracic Surg. 2009;25:28–31.
12. Ackermann J, Damrath V. Chemie und Technologie der Silicone. Herstellung und Verwendung von Siliconpolymeren Chemie. 1989;86–99.
13. Richards RB. Polyethylene-structure, crystallinity and properties. J App Chem. 2007;8:370–6.
14. Halden RU. Plastics and health risks. Ann Rev Pub Health. 2010;31:179–94.
15. Redon H. Closure under reduced atmospheric pressure of extensive wounds. Mem Acad Chir. 1954;80:394–6. http://www.carefusion.com/our-products/interventional-specialties/drainage/about-the-pleurx-drainage-system/pleurx-drainage-system.
16. Gamie JS et al. The pigtail catheter for pleural drainage: a less invasive alternative to tube thoracostomy. JSLS. 1999;3(1):57–61.
17. Laws D, Neville E, Duffy J. Pleural diseases group, standards of care committee, British thoracic society. BTS guidelines for the insertion of a chest drain. Thorax. 2003;58 Suppl 2:ii53–9.
18. Bell RL, Ovadia P, Abdullah F, Spector S, Rabinovici R. Chest tube removal: end-inspiration or end-expiration? J Trauma. 2001;50(4):674–7.
19. Aho JM, Ruparel RK, Rowse PG, Brahmbhatt RD, Jenkins D, Rivera M. Tube thoracostomy: a structured review of case reports and a standardized format for reporting complications. World J Surg. 2015;11:2691–706.
20. Wells BJ, Roberts DJ, Grondin S, et al. To drain or not to drain? Predictors of tube thoracostomy insertion and outcomes associated with drainage of traumatic hemothoraces. Injury. 2015;9:1743–8.
21. Joshi JM. Intercostal tube drainage of pleura: urosac as chest drainage bag. J Assoc Physicians India. 1996; 6:381–2.

Chapter 5
Different Drainage Systems and Philosophies

Thomas Kiefer

Recently the discussion about drainage systems and drainage philosophies was focussed on the question of "suction or no suction" with "no suction" meaning water seal. Proponents of "permanent suction therapy" are located mainly in Europe, whereas the American community promoted use of "water seal" as a separate therapy rather than being "no suction". With increasing knowledge concerning the pathophysiology of the pleural space this discussion has almost completely been brought to an end.

Different drainage systems and their drainage philosophies must be viewed in the historical context of a period of technical stagnation. Now with newer technologies, the management of the pleural space is better understood and treated appropriately.

T. Kiefer
Chefarzt Klinik für Thoraxchirurgie, Lungenzentrum Bodensee, Klinikum Konstanz, Luisenstr. 7, 78464 Konstanz, Germany
e-mail: Thomas.Kiefer@glkn.de

© Springer International Publishing Switzerland 2017
T. Kiefer (ed.), *Chest Drains in Daily Clinical Practice*,
DOI 10.1007/978-3-319-32339-8_5

5.1   Definitions

5.1.1   Water Seal

Water seal works as a check or one way valve. Fluid and air is evacuated from the chest through the drainage system into the collection canister without the ability or hazard to go backwards (Fig. 5.1).

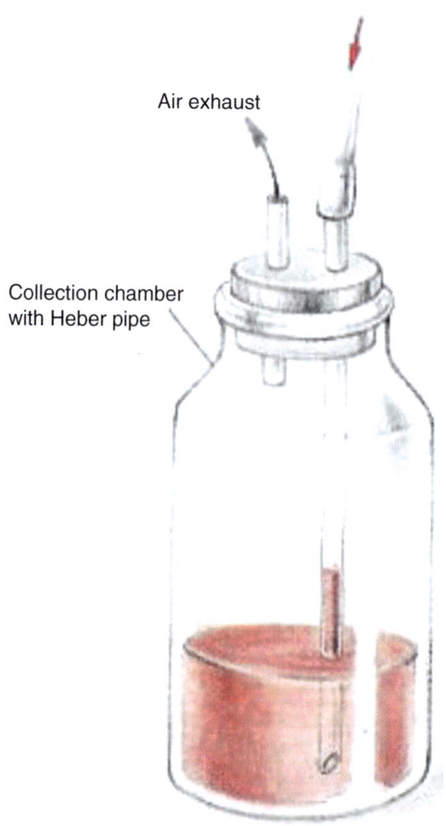

FIGURE 5.1   Water seal (From: G. Heberer, F.W. Schildberg, L. Sunder-Plassmann, I. Vogt-Maykopf Die Praxis der Chirurgie – Lunge und Mediastinum. Second edition. ISBN 3-540-19114-3, Page 191 ff)

Using a Heber-drain (see below), water seal is absolutely necessary, as the system uses an active, analogue suction source that the water seal represents. In the event of failure, an additional safety feature to prevent the patient from harm, such as a pneumothorax, is in place. In an electronic system, the check valve acts in the sense of a water seal, and is integrated into the system.

5.1.2   Heber-Drain

The Heber-drain is the classic gravity drain that works according to the so called Heber-principle using hydrostatic pressure (Fig. 5.2). When this is applied to a chest drainage system, the tubing is filled with fluid with the vertical height between chest cavity and collection canister determining the resultant subatmospheric pressure in the pleural space. In clinical practice, this means that having a patient in a bed and the canister on the floor causes a vertical height of about 60 cm. This results in a pressure in the pleural space of minus 60 cm of water.

When using a Heber-drain, it is mandatory that the collection canister is placed below the level of the chest!

A Heber-drain is always combined with a water seal component.

A Heber-drain or a water seal collection canister is without an active suction source. This system always generates a subatmospheric pressure in the pleural space dependent on the vertical height between the chest and the collection canister. This is usually a distance of 60 cm with the patient in bed with the canister on the floor causing minus 60 cm of water. It is assumed that the tubing is partially filled with fluid.

5.1.3   Bülau-Drain

The Bülau-Principle was developed by the pulmonologist Gotthard Bülau (1835–1900) in Hamburg. He used this

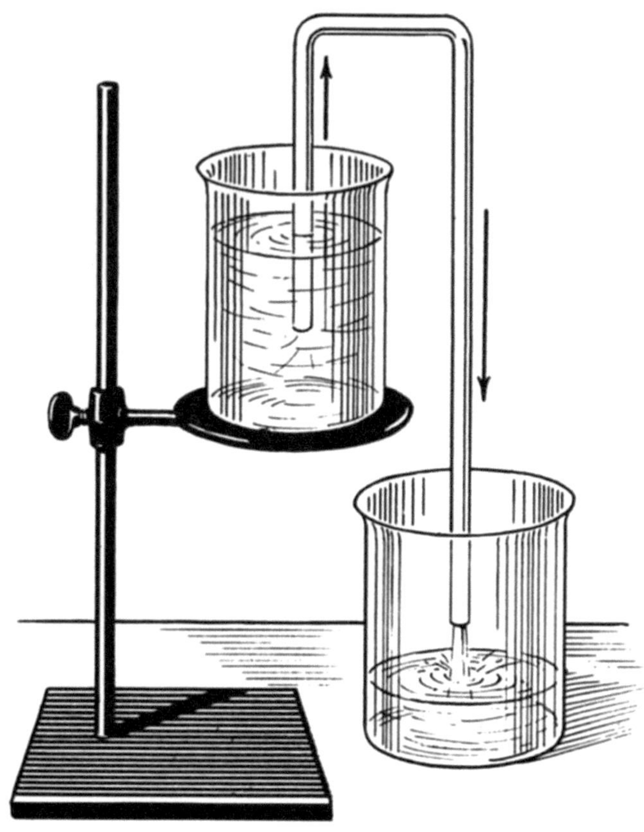

FIGURE 5.2 Heber-principle

principle for the first time in 1875 to treat a pleural empyema. The Bülau-principle is based on the application of a permanent passive suction generated by an Heber-system within a closed system (Fig. 5.3).

A Bülau-principle is a therapeutic drain using permanent passive suction generated by a Heber-drain rather than a particular catheter or drainage system.

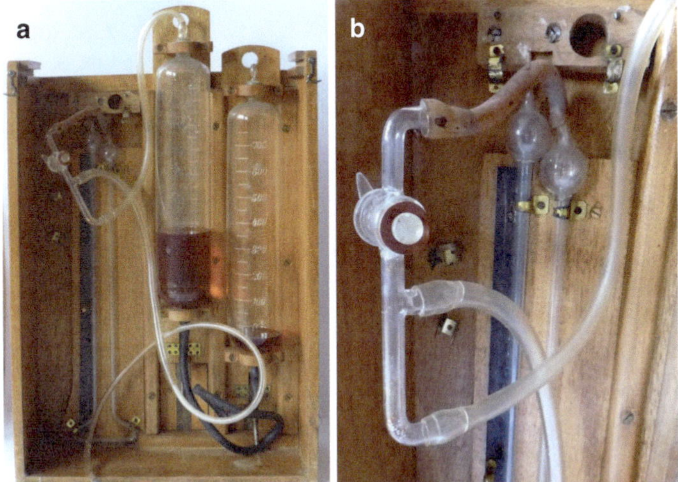

FIGURE 5.3 (**a**) and (**b**) Bülau-Drain-System

5.1.4 Monaldi-Drain

Vincenzo Monaldi (1899–1969) first described chest tube insertion in the second intercostal space in the midclavicular line. According to the author, this localization should be avoided as the intercostal spaces in that area are very narrow leading to pain when chest a tube is placed there. The skin incision is also in a very visible region where scars can develop keloids and are unsightly. There was a drain used for the therapy treatment of pulmonary abscesses named the "Monaldi-drain".

5.1.5 Heimlich-Valve

A Heimlich-valve (Fig. 5.4) is a check or one way valve that was named after the American physician Henry Heimlich who was born in 1920. Due to the integrated rubber lip in

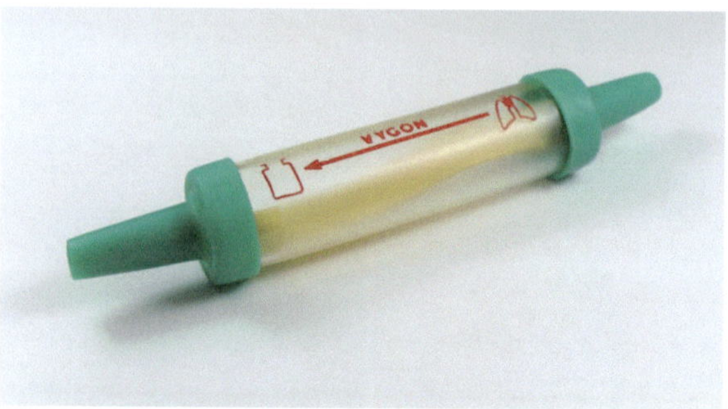

FIGURE 5.4 Heimlich-valve

device, fluid and air are allowed to escape from the chest into the collection bag. Fluid and air are unable to reflux in the opposite direction as the rubber lip will collapse making such transit impossible.

Heimlich-valves can be used if there is a relatively small but persistent air leak in a mobile patient with minimal fluid production. In emergency situations such as a tension pneumothorax), the Heimlich-valve is a safe and simple but effective tool. In Germany it is part of the standard equipment in rescue vans.

In German speaking regions, the Heimlich-valve is used less often than in the American world as the length of stay due to many non-medical reasons is much shorter compared to Europe or Germany.

5.2 Drainage Systems

Before discussing different drainage systems, one must consider some basic requirements that a clinicians will ask for today in such a system. The following criteria must be fulfilled:

1. The system is simple and safe
2. The different components are simple, easy, and fast to assemble
3. The system can be used for all chest drain indications

4. Mobility of the patient is guaranteed
5. The system is reliable
6. The system is quiet
7. The system is light weight
8. The system is cost effective

This list includes safety issues [1–5], aspects of patient's comfort [6, 7] as well as economic points that have become more and more important.

In regards to #3, the possibility of ubiquitous use is also a safety issue as the use of a single system in a hospital will increase patient's safety due to familiarity and availability.

5.2.1   One-Chamber-System

A one chamber system consists of the collection canister (Fig. 5.5) that in convention includes a water seal component with the possibility to evacuate air (actively or passively) towards the atmosphere. In the new electronic devices, the collection chamber is directly connected to the suction source where a check-valve is integrated.

In theory, the majority of indications for chest drainage can be fulfilled with a one chamber system. Such a system can be used as a Heber-drain or in combination with an active suction source. There is a limitation with conventional systems that include a collection canister and suction source from different suppliers when there is a huge air leak.

When using a one chamber system such as a Heber-drain (no active suction), the fluid must be manually milked down to the canister because there is a potential for air to not be able to escape depending on the pressure gradient. Remember the difference in height between the canister and patient determines this pressure. This could mean that the patient would not be able to evacuate air just by breathing and/or coughing which could cause a pneumothorax and possibly subcutaneous emphysema.

The occurrence of a so called "siphon-effect" (see below) must also be prevented.

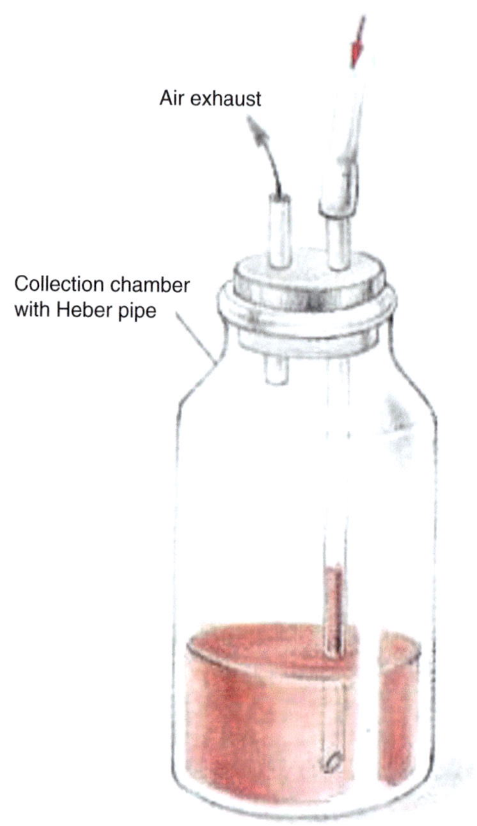

FIGURE 5.5 One-chamber-system (From: G. Heberer, F.W. Schildberg, L. Sunder-Plassmann, I. Vogt-Maykopf Die Praxis der Chirurgie – Lunge und Mediastinum. Second edition. ISBN 3-540-19114-3, Page 191 ff)

Modern electronic systems in which the canister is integrated into the system do not have these same limitations as they are in effect a two chamber system. This is achieved with the geometry of the tubing and the connections that are in place. When entering the system, fluid and air are separated with fluid into the collection chamber and air evacuated through the system into the atmosphere.

5.2.2   Two-Chamber-System

Two chamber systems were developed to prevent foam formation which is due to protein rich surfactant seen in patients with a large air leak. There can be a lot of foam in a one chamber system with water seal which can make the observation and quantity of an air leak more difficult or even impossible to see. The two chamber system also prevents that from rising up in the tubing towards the patient.

Fluid and air are directed via tubing to the collection canister where fluid falls due to gravity. The air moves forward to the second canister that has the water seal and then is evacuated either actively or passively (Fig. 5.6).

5.2.3   Multi-Chamber-System

Multi chamber systems, mostly three chamber, were developed during the time where there were no mobile suction sources available. The only suction source available in a hospital was wall suction delivered by the so called central vacuum with a pressure of minus 100 cm of water. In earlier days there had been no pressure relief valves available to decease the negative pressure to a therapeutic level.

In addition to the two chamber systems, a third chamber, the water-vacuometer chamber, was linked. This closed chamber was filled with water where a pipe was plugged in. The deeper the pipe depth, the bigger the subatmospheric pressure generated in the pleural space (Fig. 5.7).

In the very beginning these systems had been created by adding a third glass bottle. These systems were very bulky and accident laden. Eventually, commercial suppliers developed and sold these systems. Thanks to modern technical possibili-

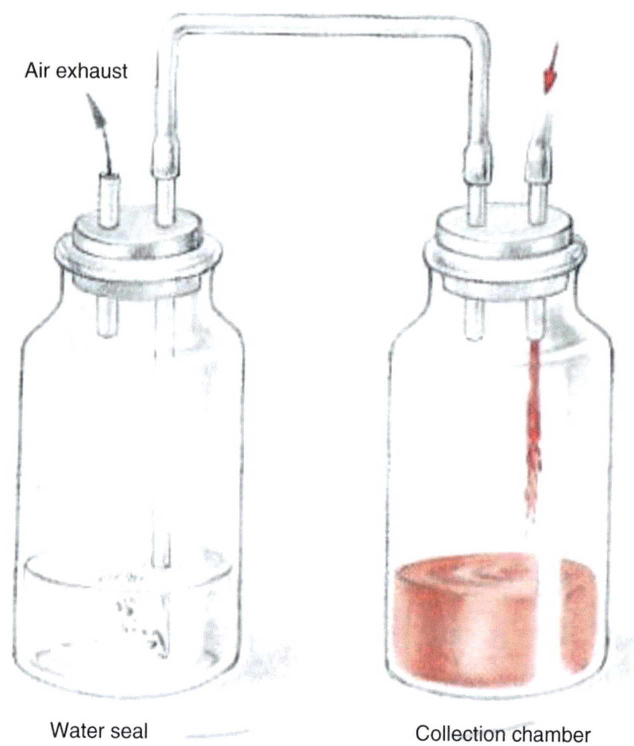

FIGURE 5.6 Two-chamber-system (From: G. Heberer, F.W. Schildberg, L. Sunder-Plassmann, I. Vogt-Maykopf Die Praxis der Chirurgie – Lunge und Mediastinum. Second edition. ISBN 3-540-19114-3, Page 191 ff)

ties, there is really not a need for these systems anymore. Most of the commercially available multi-chamber-systems need high flows (up to 20 l/min) to be able to work due to their mechanics.

Multi chamber systems that are commercially available today date back to earlier systems that were needed due to a lack of technical alternatives. Today there is no more need for such systems as superior alternatives exist.

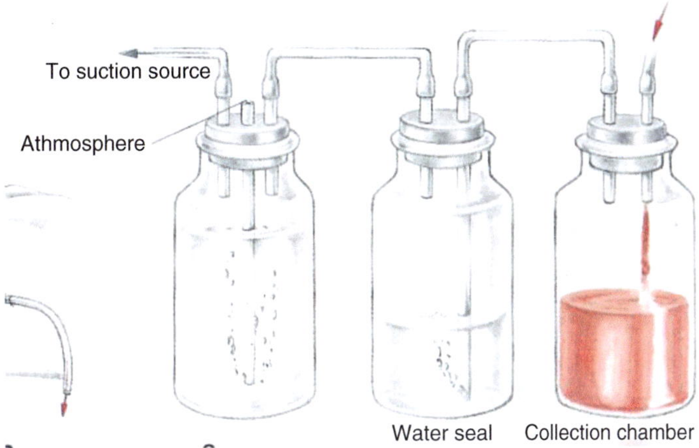

Figure   5.7 Three-chamber-system   (From: G.   Heberer, F.W. Schildberg, L. Sunder-Plassmann, I. Vogt-Maykopf Die Praxis der Chirurgie – Lunge und Mediastinum. Second edition. ISBN 3-540-19114-3, Page 191 ff)

5.2.4   Electronic Systems

Over the recent past, electronic systems (Fig. 5.8) have become commercially available which allow the collection chamber to be integrated into the system. This has allowed for minimization of the system which has aided in patient mobilization. The addition of observation software has made possible the generation of objective data concerning air leaks and fluid production for real time data collection. The monitor is as close as possible to the pleural space as it is located in the connecter between catheter and the system's tubing (Fig. 5.9).

The tubing used in these electronic systems is made of a double lumen which allows for the separation of air and fluid. The thinner tube of double lumen tubing is used for pressure measurement in the pleural cavity. In an ideal word, although technically possible but not currently commercially available,

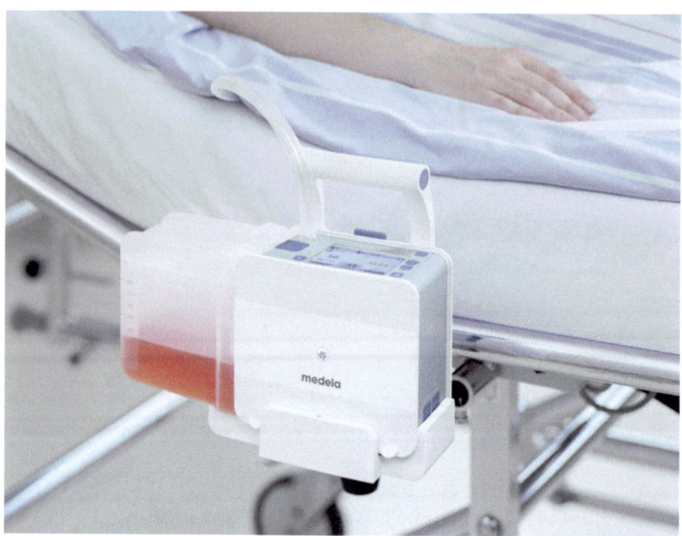

FIGURE 5.8 Electronic system (Illustration printed with permission from Medela)

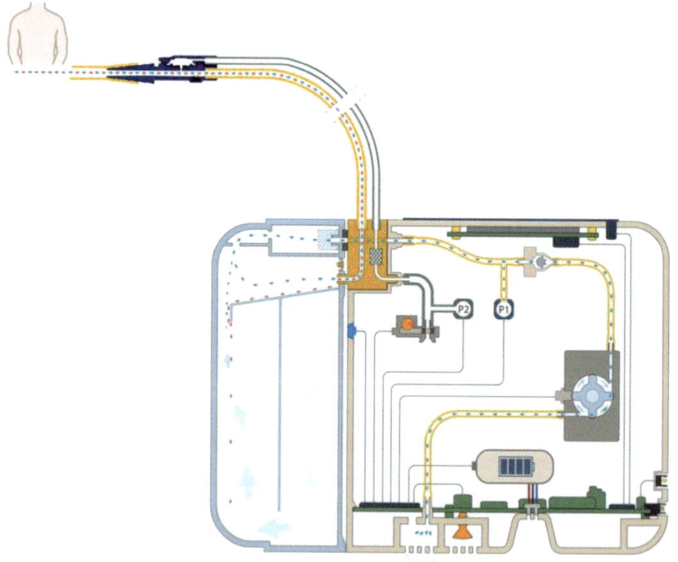

FIGURE 5.9 Thopaz Medela (Photograph printed with permission from Medela)

the pressure measurements would be from the intrapleural cavity. Experimental studies show that the data received next to the pleural space comes quite close to measurements in the pleural space [1].

With the ability to acquire, store, and interpret objective data from these electronic systems, is has become apparent that healing is dynamic process. Numerous studies have shown that using this information, the chest drainage time after anatomic resections can be shortened by 1 day on average [2–5].

Measurement of an air leak (alveolo-pleural fistula) follows the "paddle-wheel principle". This means that according to the rotation speed of the integrated paddle-wheel (Fig. 5.9) a mathematical algorithm is able to calculate very precisely the amount of air that is being drained. This is represented on the display as the flow in ml/min. After one hour, a graph is visible showing the course of the leak over the time based upon this data.

Another very important aspect of the measurement is the fact that objective data is generated which is not dependent on the observation and interpretation of the engaged staff. It has been shown [6, 7] that discrepancies in evaluation of the clinical course are significantly lower when using an electronic system compared to conventional systems.

Monitoring and alarm features increase the safety of the treatment and reduce the work load of the nursing staff [8].

It is important that such a system is not just a "pump" applying "permanent suction" to the pleural space. In fact, the pleural space is monitored and the system intervenes only as needed to achieve the desired value. This is shown in that the "pump" in the system has only 90 min of drainage time during the 2.5 days after an uncomplicated lobectomy.

5.3   Drainage Philosophies

There are a couple of definitions that are used in the clinical setting that are sometimes used in an incorrect way and therefore need clarification.

5.3.1 Negative Pressure

From a physical standpoint "negative pressure" does not exist! This is intended to express a difference in pressure between two spaces and in these cases means between the atmosphere and the pleural space. To be correct this means that were are referring to a subatmospheric pressure in the pleural space rather than "negative pressure" [9].

5.3.2 Vacuum

Very often it is said that a "vacuum is applied" or "a vacuum is generated". The precise definition of "vacuum" is a space with zero pressure (i.e. the universe) [9]. This is a situation that we do not achieve with our drainage systems!

5.3.3 Active vs. Passive Suction

The wording "passive suction" was widely used when referring to the drainage of air and fluid as the intrappleural pressure is higher than the atmospheric pressure. According to the consensus paper from 2011 [10] we are now talking about "no external suction".

To drain in an active manner, a subatmospheric pressure at the tip of the catheter has to be generated. According to the consensus paper [10] active suction refers to external suction.

5.3.4 Regulated vs. Unregulated Suction

Old fashioned drainage systems that were commercially available allowed for regulation of suction in the system, but did not suction subatmospheric pressure in the pleural space!

Regulated suction in the canister means unregulated suction in the pleural space. Water seal is always an uncontrolled, unregulated, potentially unknown suction in the pleural space.

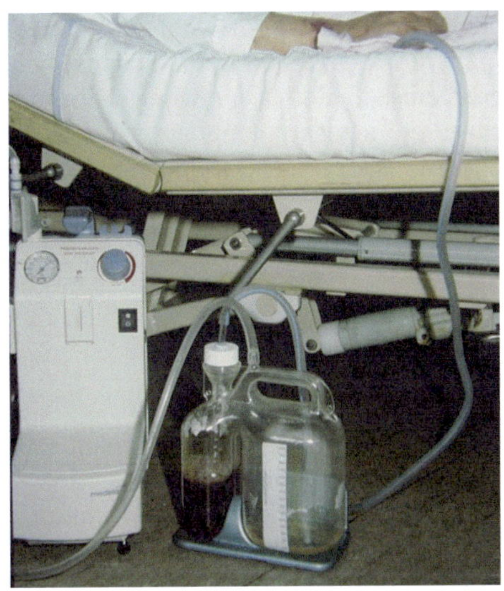

FIGURE 5.10 Siphon

5.3.5   *Siphon*

As the tubing creates a sagging loop filled with fluid (Fig. 5.10) the subatmospheric pressure that results in the pleural space is reduced due to the vertical height of that fluid column. Using a drainage system with an active suction source set on minus 20 cm of water and with the fluid in the syphon rising up 10 cm as well, the resulting pressure in the pleural space is just minus 10 cm of water! In actuality the siphon effect will be more than 10 cm of water. With all of these analogous systems, we don't know the exact subatmospheric pressure that results in the pleural space because we only know the pressure set in the system.

On the other hand, when using a Heber-drain (permanent passive suction), the patient lying in bed with the canister on the floor generates a subatmospheric pressure in the pleura space of 60 cm of water. This is due to the 60 cm of difference in vertical height between floor where the canister sits and where the patient is positioned in the hospital bed.

These problems do not occur when using an electronic system because the measurements are taken as near as possible to the pleural space at the connection between the tubing and catheter. This is the reason why the electronic system works correctly irrespective of where it is placed (on the floor or above the chest).

5.3.6 Drainage Philosophies

Traditionally there were two drainage philosophies which included permanent suction and no suction. There are numerous studies [11–14] with regard to the question whether suction is harmful or helpful in treating air leaks. These studies and the author's own clinical experience have shown that in most cases the decision has to be made in an individualized fashion. The components that help in the decision making process include the patient's underlying disease, status of the lung tissue ("normal", fibrotic, emphysematous), timing, and the surgical procedure.

The mindset of "either or" is antiquated. Thanks to modern electronic drainage systems, there is a better understanding of what is going on the pleural space. This knowledge supports an individualized approach to the intrapleural space.

The goal of chest tube therapy is to restore the normal physiological status of the intrapleural space.

5.3.7 Management of the Pleural Space

Today we are talking about the management of the pleural space. Clinicians have tried applying different subatmosheric pressure settings in patients with different anatomic resections (right upper lobectomy vs. left lower lobectomy). However, until today, the clinical relevance of these rather theoretical considerations had not been proven [15].

With the advent of the electronic drainage systems, we are now able to monitor the pleural space. The system only intervenes as when the measured value and the set differ. The system generates a subatmospheric pressure thus evacuating air from the pleural space as long as the set value is reached.

As you can see, the discussion is no longer "suction or no suction". Instead the discussion is more about which system configuration is an optimal solution for an individual patient. The hope is that this discussion will allow for the safest and most efficient therapeutic algorithms to be generated for future patients.

Literature

1. Miserocchi G, Negrini D. Pleural space: pressure and fluid dynamics. In: Crystal RG, West JB, editors. THE LUNGE, Scientific Foundations. New York: Raven Press; 1997. p. 1217–25 (Chapter 88).
2. Varela G, Jiménez MF, Novoa NM, Aranda JL. Postoperative chest tube management: measuring air leak using an electronic device decreases variability in the clinical practice. Eur J Cardiothorac Surg. 2009;35:28–31.
3. Brunelli A, Salati M, Refai M, Di Nunzio L, Xiumé F, Sabbatini A. (2010). Evaluation of a new chest tube removal protocol using digital air leak monitoring after lobectomy: a prospective randomised trial. Eur J Cardio-thorac Surg. 2010;37:56–60.
4. Mier JM, Molins L, Fibla JJ. The benefits of digital air leak assessment after pulmonary resection: Prospective and comparative study. Cir Esp. 2010;87(6):385–9.
5. Pompili C, Detterbeck F, Papagionnopoulos K, Sihoe A, Vachlas K, Maxfield MW, et al. Multicenter international randomized comparison of objective and subjective outcomes between electronic and traditional chest drainage systems. Ann Thorac Surg. 2014;98: 490–7.
6. Cerfolio RJ, Bryant AS. The quantification of postoperative air leaks. Mult Man Cardiothorac Sur. 2009. doi:10.1510/mmcts.2007.003129.
7. McGuire AL, Petrich W, Maziak DE, Shamji FM, Sundaresan SR, Seely AJE, et al. Digital versus analogue pleural drainage phase 1: prospective evaluation of interobserver reliability in the

assessment of pulmonary air leaks. Interact CardioVasc Thorac Surg. 2015;21:403–8.

8. Danitsch D. Benefits of digital thoracic drainage systems. Benefits of digital thoracic drainage systems. Nursing Times 13 Mar 2012;108:11.

9. Linder A. Thoraxdrainagen und Drainagesystem – Moderne Konzepte UNI-MED Verlag. 2014.

10. Brunelli A, Beretta E, Cassivi SD, Cerfolio RJ, Detterbeck F, Kiefer T, et al. Consensus definitions to promote an evidence-based approach to management oft he pleural space. A collaborative proposal by ESTS, AATS. STS GTSC Eur J Cardio-thorac Surg. 2011;40(2011):291–97.

11. Balfour-Lynn IM et al. BTS guidelines fort he management of pleural infection in children. Thorax. 2005;60(Suppl I):i1–i21.

12. Sammi A, Critchley A, Dunning J. Should chest drains be put on suction or not following pulmonary lobectomy? Inter CardioVasc Thorac Surg. 2006;5:275–8.

13. Merritt RE, Singhal S, Shrager JB. Evidence-based suggestions for management of air leaks. Thorac Surg Clin. 2010;20:435–48. doi:10.1016/j.thorsurg.2010.03.005.

14. Pompeili C, Xiumè F, Hristova R, Salati M, Refai M, Milton R, et al. Regulated drainage reduces the incidence of recurrence after uniportal video-assisted thoracoscopic bullectomy for primary spontaneous pneumothorax: a propensity case-matched comparison of regulated and unregulated drainage. Eur J Cardiothorac Surg. 2015;49:1–5. doi:10.1093/ejcts/ezr056.

15. Refai M, Brunelli A, Varela G, Novoa N, Pompili C, Jimenez MF, et al. The values of intrapleural pressure before removal of chest tube in non-complicated pulmonary lobectomies. Eur J Cardiothorac Surg. 2012;41:1–3. doi:10.1093/ejcts/ezr056.

Chapter 6
Inserting a Chest Drain: How to Do

Thomas Kiefer

This chapter refers only to the placing of a chest tube by minithoracotomy. Chest tubes placed at the end of an operation are not included here. The insertion technique of small-bore catheters is very similar to thoracocentesis and therefore is not discussed here.

Inserting a chest tube by the so called "trocar technique" is obsolete! Complications related with this technique are of concerning frequency and severity, which are not acceptable [1]. See also Chap. 7.

6.1 Localization

Localization of the skin incision and entry point for the chest tube should be chosen based on the tube indication. If a loculated effusion or an empyema has to be drained it is strongly recommended to determine the location using ultrasound.

As a general rule, insertion of a chest drain in the fourth intercostal space in the anterior midaxillary line can be used to treat many pathologies (i.e. free effusion, pneumothorax)

T. Kiefer
Chefarzt Klinik für Thoraxchirurgie, Lungenzentrum Bodensee, Klinikum Konstanz, Luisenstr. 7, 78464 Konstanz, Germany
e-mail: Thomas.Kiefer@glkn.de

© Springer International Publishing Switzerland 2017   93
T. Kiefer (ed.), *Chest Drains in Daily Clinical Practice*,
DOI 10.1007/978-3-319-32339-8_6

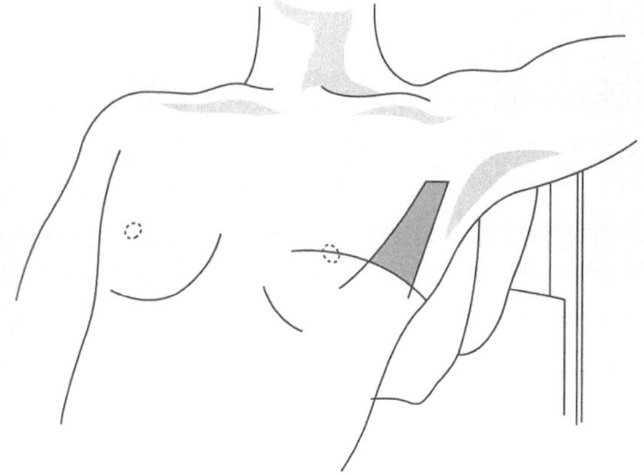

Figure 6.1 Safe triangle

The "safe triangle" refers to [2] Fig. 6.1. The fourth intercostal space is located two fingerbreaths below the nipple in men and at the submammary fold in women.

A more posteriorly located chest tube may be uncomfortable as the patient may lay on it, causing pain and kinking of the tube with subsequent clogging. In general the skin incision should not be placed posterior to the *spina iliaca anterior superior*.

If there is a need for a chest tube placed posteriorly (i.e. to drain an empyema), there should be padding placed on the chest tube to minimize discomfort and tube issues.

6.1.1 Monaldi Position

The so-called Monaldi position (V. Monaldi 1899–1969) using the second intercostal space in the midaxillary line for chest drain insertion should not be used in the author's opinion. This chest tube position was previously used for draining apical pneumothoraces. These patients are frequently young with spontaneous pneumothoraxes and the incision is in a very visible location. If there are problems with the scar, such as a keloid, it is very unsightly. Additionally the intercostal space in the location is very narrow causing more pain related to the chest tube and is another reason to avoid this access.

The again and again quoted "Bülau-Position" does not exist! Gotthard Bülau (1835–1900) neither developed a drainage system nor described localization of a skin incision for chest tube insertion. He became famous as he was the first who used the Heber principle, a passive permanent suction, (see Chap. 5) in the conservative treatment of an empyema. He used the Heber drain successfully for the first time in 1875 in a carpenter suffering from a pleural empyema and published the methods in 1891 [3].

6.1.2 *Posterior Suprascapular Access*

Posterior suprascapular access is rarely used. The indication for this placement is in a postoperative patient with pneumothorax where there are adhesions to the chest wall. If there is concern for parenchymal damage using a more "conventional" access, this could be used. One must affirm there is a real need for a chest drain in this patient with an "apical pneumothorax" with symptoms or is the chest tube just treating a stuck lung for "cosmetic" reasons on the x-ray!

The fourth intercostal space is located two fingerbreaths below the nipple in men. In women the fourth intercostal space is at the level of the submammary fold. Skin incisions should not be placed posterior of the *spina iliaca anterior superior*.

6.2   Informed Consent

Medico-legal aspects are more and more important in daily clinical work. Thus, with the exception of an emergency procedure, informed consent has to be obtained from the patient. The discussion and documentation should include:
- Indication for chest tube insertion
- Therapeutic alternatives (if present)
- Explanation of the procedure
- Potential complications
- Further clinical course

The consent must be documented in one of the commercial available forms. At least according to German law, a copy of this form has to be handed over to the patient.

6.3 Patient Positioning

It is crucial to remember that the insertion of a chest tube in many cases is an urgent or emergent procedure. This may be the first invasive for the patient after admission. The circumstances surround positioning and placement may be uncomfortable and traumatizing for the patient, which can make future interactions between patient and physician somewhat more difficult!

Patient positioning depends on the location chosen for drain insertion. The patient has to be positioned in a way that he feels comfortable, minimizes (additional) pain and in case of large effusion, dyspnea is not worsened.

Most often supine positioning will be chosen sometimes with the upper body elevated. Once the patient is in a safe and comfortable position, the arm of the side of intervention is placed next to the body or, in patients with sufficient energy and vigilance, behind the neck (Fig. 6.2).

In patients with a large effusion, lateral decubitus positioning may be helpful. The patient is stabilized with pillows. This positioning helps to prevent contaminating the surrounding area with any fluid (Fig. 6.3).

If the intention is to place a chest tube in the suprascapular location, the patient is in a seated position with the physician standing behind him.

6.4 Instruments

A procedure set that includes all requires instruments and disposables is strongly recommended. This guarantees availability of all utensils at all times. In an emergency situation such a set may save important time! Whether this set is individually composed or delivered from a manufacturer Fig. 6.4 is not the issue. By using procedure sets adherent to a SOP used in most centers today this is a supported practice.

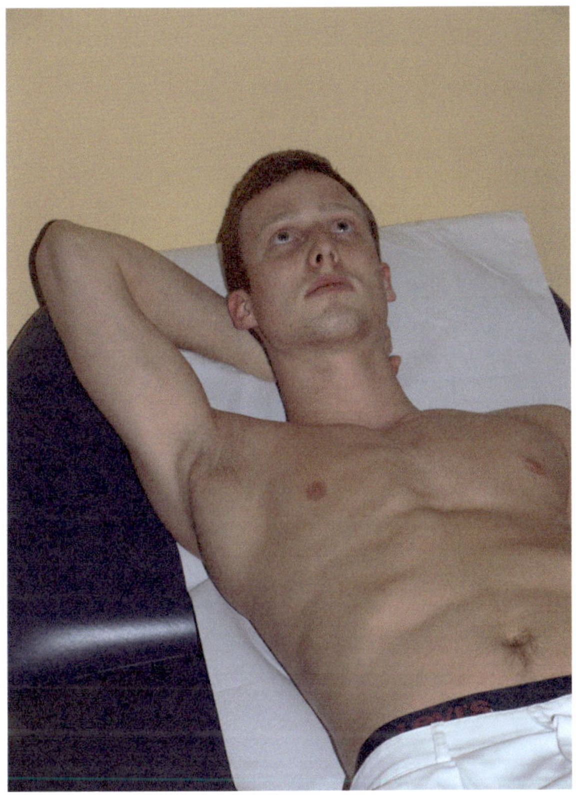

FIGURE 6.2 Supine position

6.5   Different Types of Drains

Drains can be differentiated by material, diameter, configurations (straight or angled) as well as by the presence of a second lumen for irrigation Fig. 6.5 (details see Chap. 4).

The indication for chest drain insertion determines which drain and what size diameter should be chosen. Body composition, individual preferences, and experience are other factors that should be taken into account. Table 6.1 gives an overview.

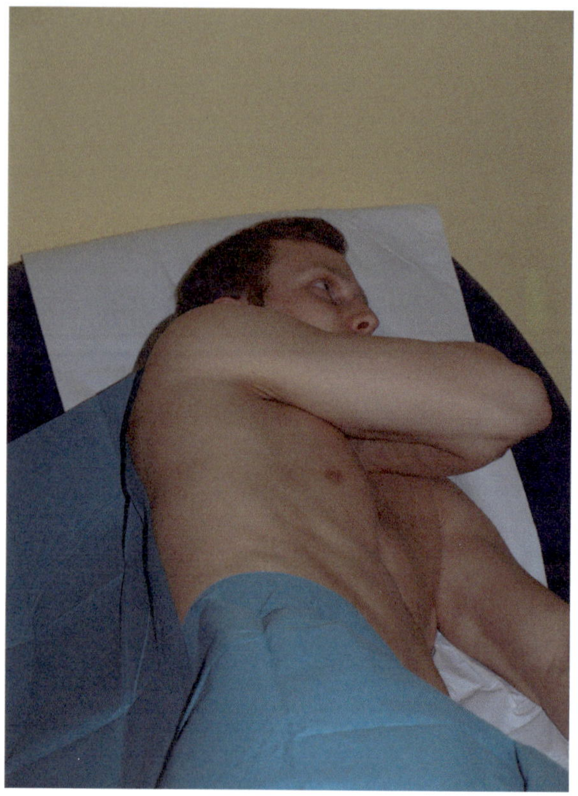

FIGURE 6.3 Lateral decubitus position

6.6   Number of Drains

One chest tube is sufficient for most drainage indications. There are studies [4] that have shown that after standard operative resections, one tube is as effective as two or more tubes. Using just one chest tube can allow for shorter drainage time (followed by a shorter length of hospital stay) and lower costs. The old law "one tube to the apex for air and one to the base for fluid" can be stopped confidently. The chest cavity is a communicating space and air and fluid can be drained by one tube.

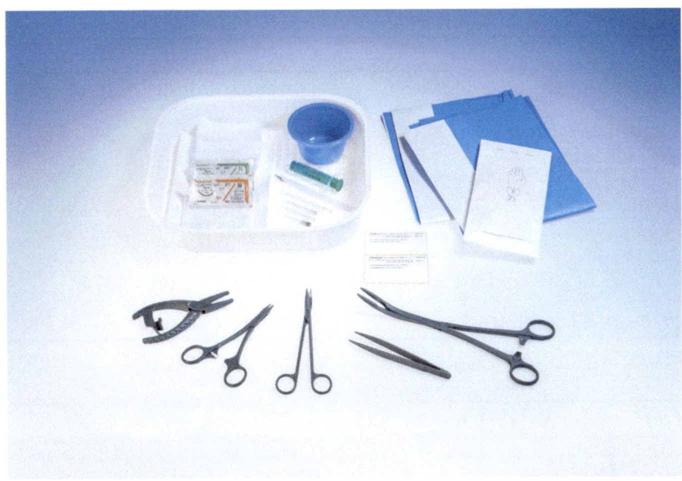

FIGURE 6.4 Procedure set for inserting a chest drain (Courtesy of B.Braun-Aesculap)

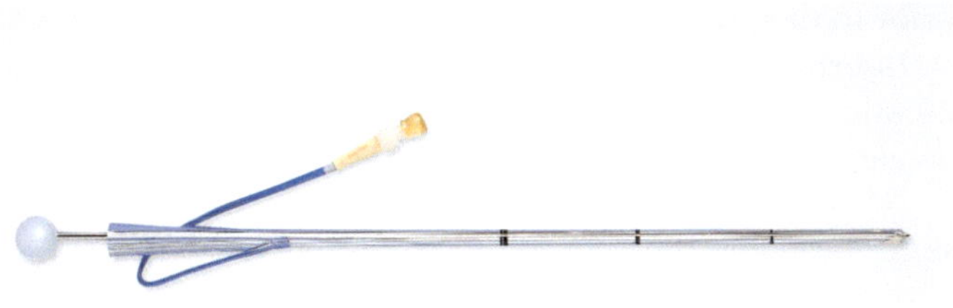

FIGURE 6.5 Drain for irrigation

There is no proof of efficacy that placing a basally directed chest tube after pleurectomy/decortication supports reexpansion of a not fully reexpanded lung. So called ring-irrigation, if indicated, does not require two tubes. With the help of an chest drain with an additional lumen for irrigation, this can be done more or less in the same way.

TABLE 6.1 Type of drain used for different indications

	Type of drain	**Diameter**
Pneumothorax	Standard drain	20 F
Pleural empyema	Irrigation drain	24–28 F
Hemothorax	Irrigation drain	24–28 F
Post-op. after standard resections	Standard drain	24 F
Post-op. after pleurodesis	Standard drain	20–24 F

6.7   How to Do

Before proceeding with chest drainage, the responsible physician needs to be absolutely sure that the correct side has been chosen! It can be beneficial to have the appropriate images in view for the procedure. When there is an effusion or pleural empyema, ultrasound should be performed immediately prior to the procedure for localization.

Insertion of a chest tube has to be performed under strict aseptic conditions: surgical gown, cap, surgical mask, and sterile gloves.

After disinfection of the hands and sterilization of the skin, local anesthetic infiltration should be performed to encompass the incision and where the securing stitch will be placed. Next the periosteum of the rib is anesthetized sufficiently as well as the underlying pleura which is very sensitive to pain. Usually 30 to a max of 40 ml of local anesthetic (1 %) should be enough in patients with a relatively normal body mass index. When obtaining the medical history prior to the procedure, one must include the question regarding intolerance to local anesthetics! The maximum dose of the drug must be kept in mind as well to prevent complications such arrhythmia or epilepsy.

When the patient is awake, nervous, or agitated it is recommended to first place the stitch that will secure the chest tube. This allows safe and quick fixation of the tube to be done very quickly thus preventing the tube from slipping out. In addition this stitch can be used to check the efficiency of the local anesthesia.

Next the incision of the skin and the subcutaneous tissue is performed with a scalpel. The incision must be wide enough allow a finger to be used for safe examination without causing pain. Further preparation is done with scissors by alternating cutting and spreading until reaching the rib, sliding over the upper edge of the rib, and then into the chest cavity.

Entering the chest cavity must always be completed above a rib! Prior to catheter insertion, a digital inspection of the chest cavity must be done, even in a complete pneumothorax, in order to prevent damage of the organs in the chest cavity, to clarify an intrathoracic position, and to exclude an intraabdominal one.

Ideally the skin incision is placed a couple of centimeters below the upper rib edge for which the chest cavity will be entered. This technique is the so called "coulisse effect" where soft tissue slides towards the chest wall, like coulisses, covering the skin incision and providing soft tissue coverage which can be helpful with very slim individuals (Fig. 6.6).

The chest tube has to be inserted with the use of minimal power. It is a strong hint that the tube is within the chest cavity when fogging is observed that is synchronous to inspiration and expiration.

If necessary the catheter is directed towards the intended position with the help of a dressing forceps. Which kind of instrument is used, if any, is not a real issue. Time and time again ideas are published which are more or less helpful [5]. The fact that none of them have been broadly established tells its own tale!

Finally the subcutaneous tissue (only in very slim individuals) and the skin is closed by a suture. When placing the stitch for the suture that will secure the tube, a large bite should be taken (Fig. 6.7). This is important in cases where the drain is in place for a long time preventing the suture from breaking through the skin. A second advantage creating such a stitch will become evident as refixation of the tube is necessary

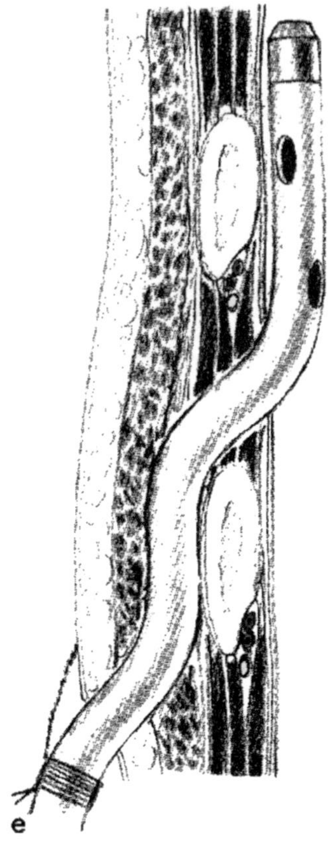

FIGURE 6.6 Coulisse effect (From: G. Heberer, F.W. Schildberg, L. Sunder-Plassmann, I. Vogt-Maykopf Die Praxis der Chirurgie – Lunge und Mediastinum. Second edition. ISBN 3-540-19114-3, Page 191 ff)

after pulling the tube back for a couple of centimeters. A new suture can be drawn through the loop of the first suture without causing pain.

Lastly another suture is placed in the middle of the remaining incision, (Fig. 6.8) the needle is cut off, and a knot is placed at the end of the string. This suture is used to close the incision after pulling the drain which is especially important in very

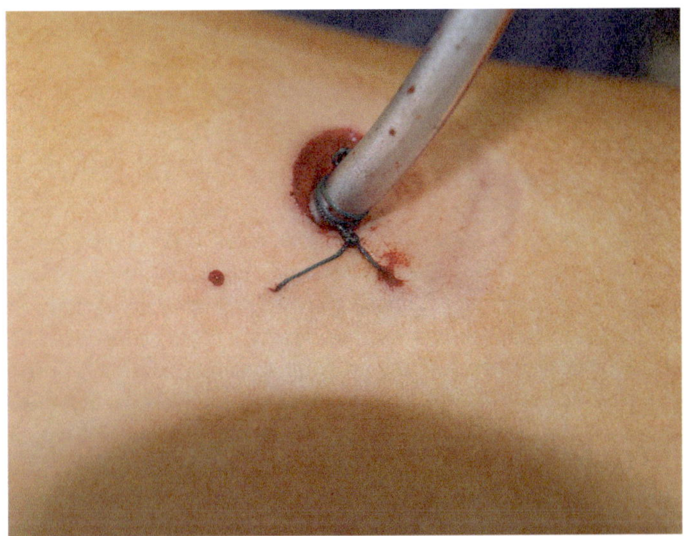

FIGURE 6.7 Fixation suture

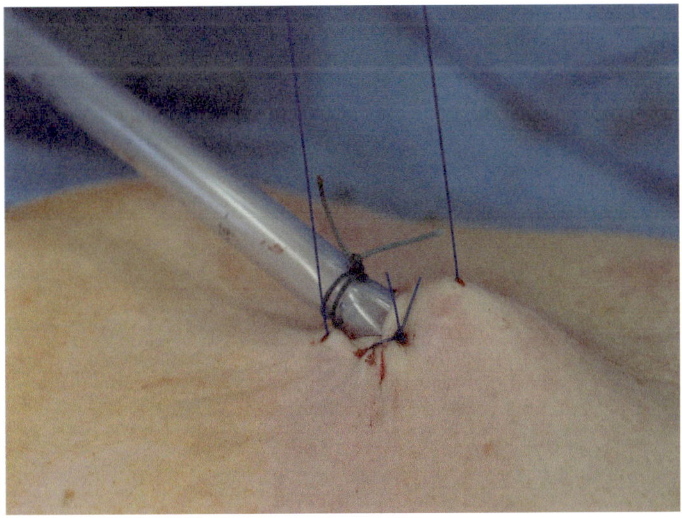

FIGURE 6.8 Additional suture for closure

slim patients (spontaneous pneumothorax!). In individuals with a higher body mass index the additional stitch is not needed.

6.7.1   Dressing

Finally the dressings are applied with y-slit compresses around the tubing, covered by "normal" compresses (10×10 cm), and an adhesive plaster. An additional fixation of the tube to the skin with a tape bridge (also called a bridle rein) is recommended to prevent tension on the fixation stitch which could cause pain (Fig. 6.9). This bridle rein also prevents the tube from moving too much to the back which could cause clogging when the patient lies on the tube. The bridle rein is not necessary when the adhesive plaster is so large as to allow the plaster to function as a bridle (Fig. 6.10). Furthermore the adhesive plaster must be applied in a way that tension is avoided in order to prevent skin injury.

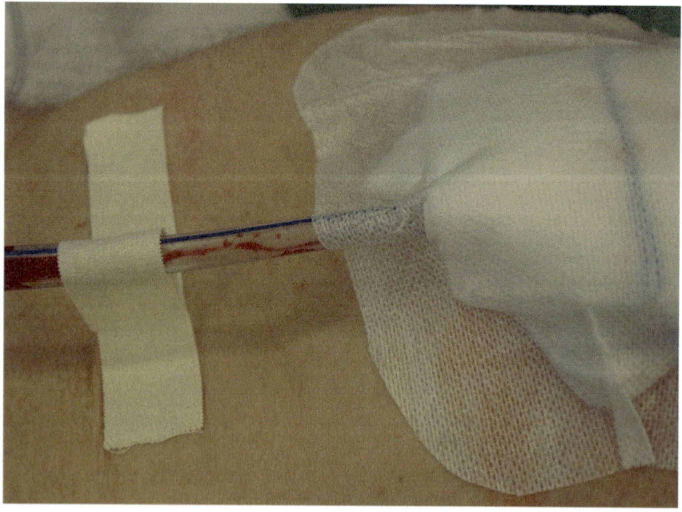

FIGURE 6.9 Adhesive plaster plus bridle rein

The tube connection may not be "secured" by a lot of plaster loops! Doing so generates a false sense of security, which may be dangerous as an observation of what is going on at the connection is no longer possible. The majority of tube connectors and adapters nowadays available are designed in a way that the connection between catheter and tubing is safe.

6.7.2   Beginning of Therapy

When the catheter is connected with the tubing of the suction system, suction shouldn't be applied suddenly. In particular this is important in huge pneumothoraces, large effusions, and when such pathologies were present for a long time period. When the lung is expanded very fast, patients usually will suffer from an intensive and nagging cough. There also seems to

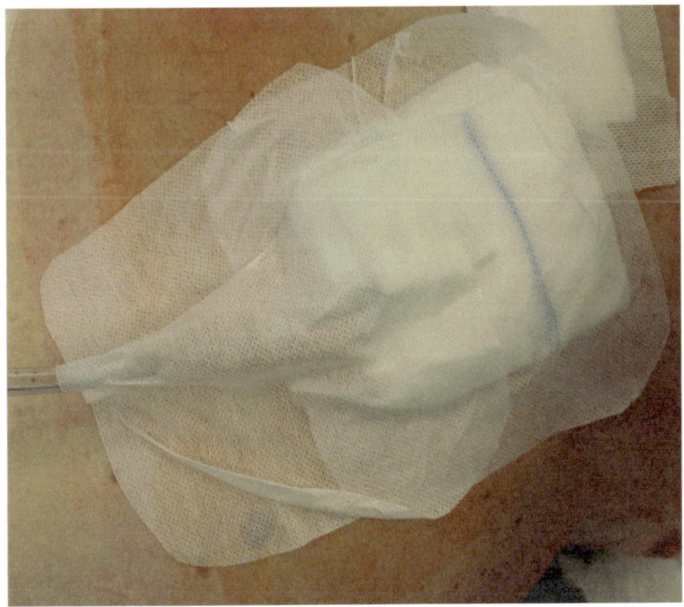

FIGURE 6.10 Adhesive plaster covering all

be a correlation between the probability of sustaining reexpansion edema when there is fast expansion of the lung (see Chap. 7). It is recommended to monitor the patient for 60 min after inserting a chest tube by measuring the oxygen saturation. After this time period the development of reexpansion edema becomes unlikely. There seems to exist a correlation between duration (more than 4 days) and degree of atelectasis (whether caused by pneumothorax or effusion) and the probability of developing reexpansion edema [6].

The catheter can be connected to the suction system and the suction activated postoperatively on the operating room table after closing the chest and finishing dressing placements.

After inserting a chest tube an x-ray is mandatory for documentation and to check proper positioning of the chest drain. This is not necessary for chest tubes placed post-operatively.

Literature

1. Balley RC. Complications of tube thoracostomy in trauma. J Accid Emerg Med. 2000;17:111–4.
2. Laws D, Neville E, Duffy J. BTS guidelines fort the insertion of a chest drain. Thorax. 2003;58:ii53–9.
3. Bülau G. Für die Heber-Drainage bei Behandlung des Empyems. Z Klin Med. 1891;18:31–4.
4. Brunelli A, Beretta E, Cassivi SD, Cerfolio RJ, Detterbeck F, Kiefer T, et al. Consensus definitions to promote an evidence-based approach to management of the pleural space. A collaborative proposal by ESTS, AATS, STS and GTSC. Eur J Card Thorac Surg. 2011;40(2011):291–7.
5. Katballe N, Moeller LB, Olesen WH, Litzer MM, Andersen G, Nekrasas V, et al. A novel device for accurate chest tube insertion: a randomized controlled trial. Eur J Cardiothorac Surg. 2015;48:893–8.
6. Rozeman J, Yellin A, Simansky DA, Shiner RJ. Re-expansion pulmonary oedema following spontaneous pneumothorax. Respir Med. 1996;90:235–8.

Chapter 7
Complications of Chest Drain Insertion and Management

Jan Volmerig

"Each mistake seems to be unbelievably stupid, as others made the mistake." (Georg Christoph Lichtenberg)

7.1 Introduction

Chest drainage and thoracocentesis represent a colorful medical mosaic in which many variables are involved:
- Experience and training status of the person performing the procedure [13, 16]
- The procedure indication: elective, palliative, urgent, or emergent
- A short term single use, a temporary intervention, or a permanent treatment with a chest drain
- Drainage of fluids with different viscosity and/or air
- Tube variations: material, diameter, shape, and number of holes

J. Volmerig
Klinik für Thoraxchirurgie, Ev. Krankenhausgemeinsxchaft Herne
Castrop-Rauxel gGmbH,
Hordeler Straße 7-9, 44651 Herne, Germany
e-mail: e.hecker@evk-herne.de

© Springer International Publishing Switzerland 2017
T. Kiefer (ed.), *Chest Drains in Daily Clinical Practice*,
DOI 10.1007/978-3-319-32339-8_7

- The therapy chosen in regard to set pressure and duration of treatment
- The procedure itself: aspiration, Seldinger-technique, trocar drain, blunt preparation
- Location for intervention: preclinical [43, 51], emergency department, intervention room, ICU, OR [8]
- Patient factors: body mass index, age, sex, comorbidities, and additional injuries

Each of these factors has an influence on the insertion of a chest drain and/or handling the drain and the associated risks. Complication rates related to these factors have been reviewed in retrospective and case studies and thus are not really comparable. Complication rates of up to 44 % have been reported [3, 34, 35].

Complications during insertion of a chest tube and subsequent management occur in up to 44 % of patients.

What conclusions can be made because of this data? How can complications be 100 % avoided? Is the "one and only one" SOP fulfilling all requirements?

One important question is: "How well do we train our young colleagues?" [3, 13, 16]

There are multiple approaches in regard to procedure technique and treatment strategy. Each type of pleural intervention has its own potential complications as well as strategies to avoid these complications. In this overview, the potential complications are discussed according to organ affected as well as some general technical considerations. The goal is to give an overview in order to provide the acting person with a case adapted risk profile in order to avoid pitfalls. To guarantee successful intervention and treatment, it is mandatory to review and analyze the entire clinical situation.

7.2   General Considerations

7.2.1   *Patient Related Framework*

Do we have to perform a diagnostic or therapeutic procedure? What is the best way to describe the clinical situation to the patient? Is there an elective, emergent, or (potentially) life threatening indication? Do therapeutic alternatives exist? Is the intervention a "cosmetic" fix for the X-ray? The underlying diagnostic information: is it valid and significant enough or should additional work up be done? Are there relevant comorbidities that could affect the procedure and treatment? Are there anatomical findings related to the underlying disease, trauma, or previous surgery? Has the patient's identity and correct side been verified and double checked? Has informed consent been obtained for the procedure and is corresponding documentation complete?

7.2.2   Aspects Concerning the Physician

Is my training and experience adequate? Is there support next door by a senior or someone on call? Do I have sufficient resources and support staff? Do I need help from others (anesthesia)? Is the chosen procedure adequate? Am I prepared for the management of potential complications?

7.2.3   Framework Concerning Room and Materials

Is the room adequate in regard to the expected findings (prehospital, emergency department, intervention room, ICU, OR)? Are all needed instruments available including less frequently utilized ones? Is it possible to assess the postinterventional findings? Is the postinterventional care guaranteed?

7.2.4   Imaging/Localization of the Drain

Pleural intervention as well as the choice of drain location is dependent on the indication for the procedure. This is the reason why the medical history, all available information, and imaging need to be reviewed. Imaging may consist of a x-ray, ultrasound, and/or CT scan. Analysis of the imaging should include such questions as: is there an inflammatory rind or a tumor? Is the thoracic anatomy normal? Are there rib fractures and where are they located?

Imaging (ultrasound, chest xray, CT scan, or a combination of these modalities) is needed to delineate patient anatomy and disease before performing any pleural intervention. This also confirms the correct side for treatment.

The choice of intervention location is many times located in the subaxillary "safe triangle" [18]. The assistance of ultrasound can aid in accessing the chest and may add valuable information [46]. After positioning of the patient for chest drain insertion, ultrasound may provide visualization and the added safety needed to be able to push harder or be more aggressive (i.e. powerful "push" though a thick pleura in an empyema). When an aspiration prior to chest drain placement

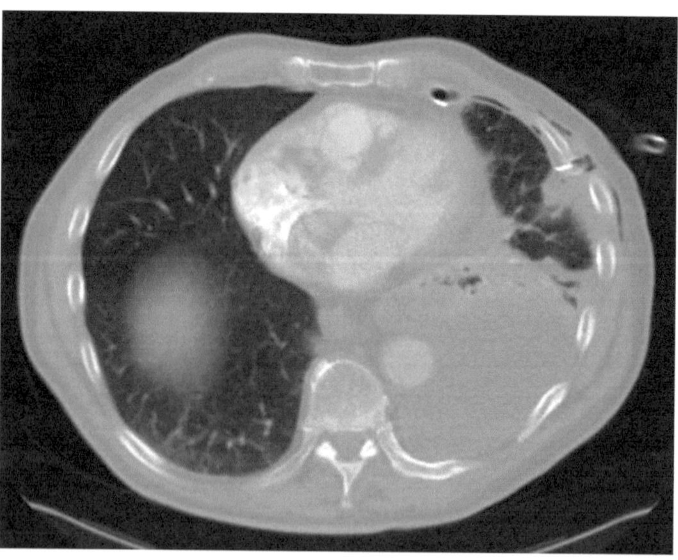

Incorrect placement of a chest drain 1

(without real time imaging) encounters blood, one may misinterpret the puncture of a blood vessel with a hemothorax. Further hints concerning imaging will be discussed in regard to specific potential complications below.

Even when chest drain placement has been performed according to intrathoracic findings, "special" topographic localization is rarely required. One should assess the potential future need for additional therapy when deciding on the diameter of the tube. Drains that are placed very posteriorly may initially have a sufficient therapeutic effect but can lose efficiency as the patient leans on it (kinking), adding pain and potential infection risk. There should always be a discussion with the patient before any procedure concerning the current disease, indication, risks/benefits, and therapeutic alternatives as issues can occur such as pain due to access-related trauma to the musculature.

The complication rates and their severity after drain insertion (particularly the so called Trocar drains) are well studied [34]. This textbook recommends and therefore explains the blunt dissection technique for the placement of a chest drains as a result of these studies.

The use of trocar drains is associated with a significant increase in complications and should therefore be avoided.

7.3   Technical Problems When Inserting a Drain

7.3.1   When a trocar drain is used, there is an increased rate of incorrect placement in an extrathoracic or subcutaneous position [24] due to the drain gliding off the ribs. The frequency of misplaced drains can be reduced by using the blunt insertion technique.

7.3.2   The placement of the chest tube may become more difficult if the chest wall is unstable due to several rib fractures or if rib segments are missing. When placing

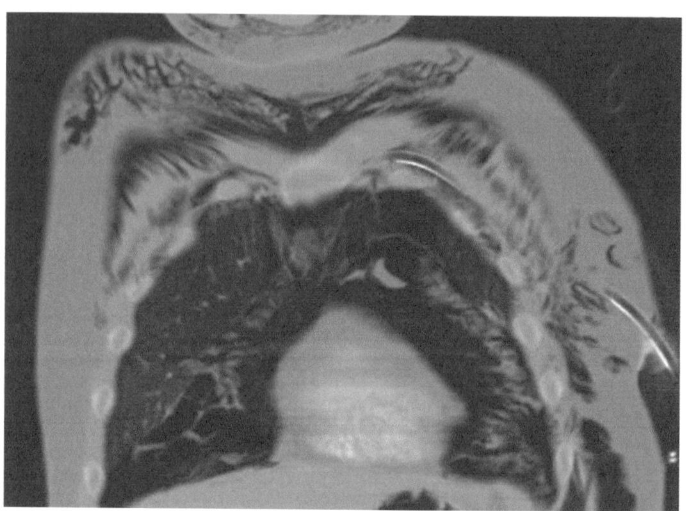

False placement of a chest drain 2

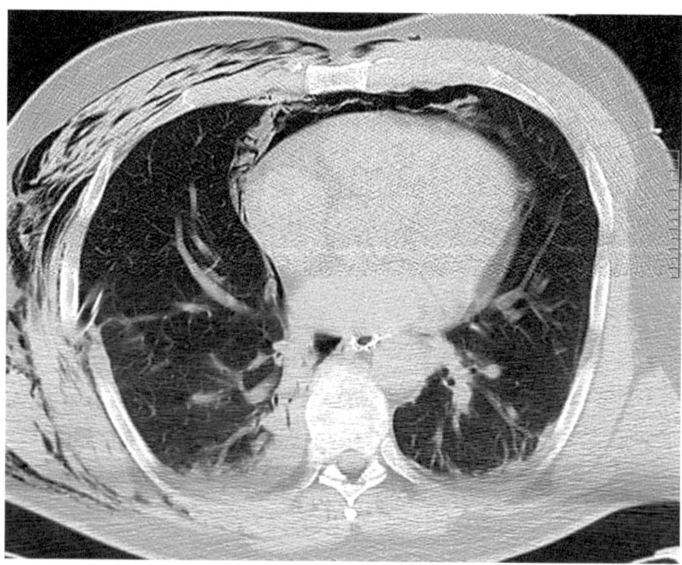

False placement of a chest drain 3

a chest drain for a traumatic indication, special attention to the imaging is crucial to avoid placing the tube next to jagged bone. This could result in cutting of the tube or persistant pain that is difficult to treat.

7.3.3 Subcutaneous emphysema can range from a discrete radiological finding to annoyance of the patient, to massive swelling causing impairment of respiratory mechanics and pacemaker malfunction [25]. Emphysema can be caused by:

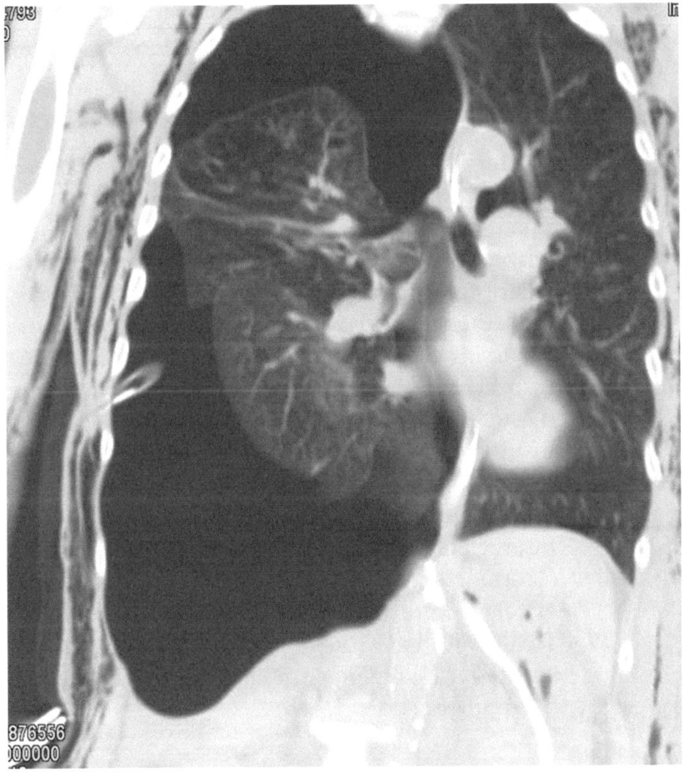

Tension pneumothorax due to clamping

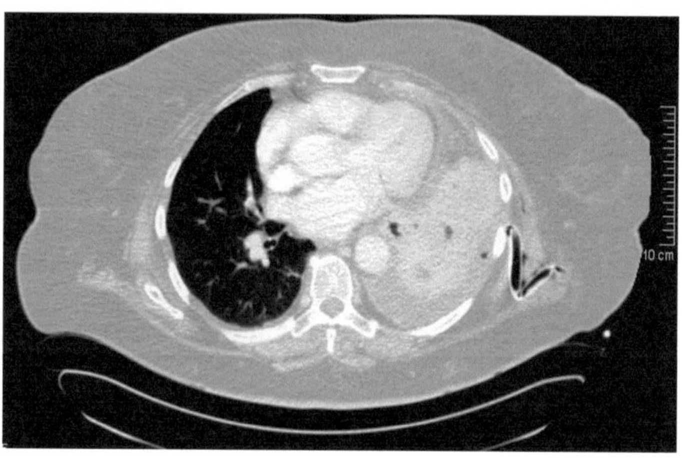

False placement of a chest drain 4

Pulmonary leakage with a mismatch of "produced" air and drainage capacity (i.e. in patients on the ventilator.

- Disproportionate large incision in the parietal pleura allowing air from the chest cavity to pass into the intercostal and subcutaneous tissue bypassing the tube.
- Insufficient placement of the intrapleural drain (i.e. interlobar)
- Insufficient placement of the chest tube where the sentinel hole is not within the chest cavity (i.e. hole in the subcutaneous tissues)
- Insufficient suction capacity due to kinked tubes (subcutaneous or extrathoracic, "forgotten"clamps) or clogged drains (blood, fibrin, tissue) [38]. Treatment is based on the removal of the obstacle(s), insertion of additional drain(s), or modification of the drainage strategy.

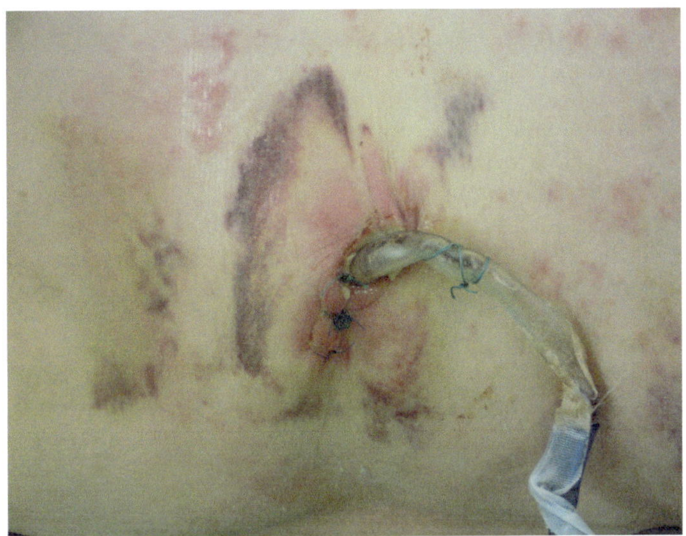

Insufficient fixation of a drain

Nasal or oral oxygen administration may accelerate absorption of subcutaneous emphysema. Procedures to relieve emphysema, such as transdermal aspiration or subcutaneous drain placement, are infrequently necessary.

7.3.4   Insufficient fixation of the drain and/or scaling of the incision can lead to skin irritation, pain, and poor efficiency of the drain. Also the development of wound infections and pleural empyemas are promoted. Daily dressing changes and wound evaluation is mandatory to diagnose an infection or any loosening of the tube fixation as early as possible. Drain dislocation, intrathoracic erosion, air leaks, and moist wound conditions may be prevented using tight suture techniques and nonabsorbable sutures.

7.4   Injuries Specific to an Organ

Not all somatic complications are avoidable when performing invasive procedures. Nevertheless a meticulous review of the clinical situation, imaging, and the patient related anatomy is mandatory. An individualized approach to any technical procedure minimizes potential risks. In the following chapters complications are discussed as they correspond to particular anatomical findings.

7.4.1   *Injuries of the Chest Wall*

Injuries to the intercostal arteries can cause life threatening bleeding [37]. Although the communicating posterior intercostal arteries arise from the aorta and the anterior intercostal arteries arise from the internal mammary arteries this by no means ensures that they run as expected in the *sulcus costalis* at the lower edge of the ribs. With advanced age, the arteries descend further inferiorly towards the intercostal space. This lower positioning is pronounced in the area near the paravertebrals (4 cm) with increasing tendency towards the lateral position (9 cm) and must be taken into consideration in all diagnostic and therapeutic aspirations in elderly patients [54].

With increasing age, the intercostal arteries (in particular posterior and lateral) no longer run in the *sulcus costalis* but may be located in the intercostal space and thus can be harmed when entering the chest through the intercostal space.

There are anatomical variations where collateral arteries at the lateral chest wall (mainly between the 8th and 11th intercostal spaces) cover two to three intercostal spaces. This is also seen inferiorly/superiorly at the fourth to seventh intercostal spaces on the right side [11, 23, 52].

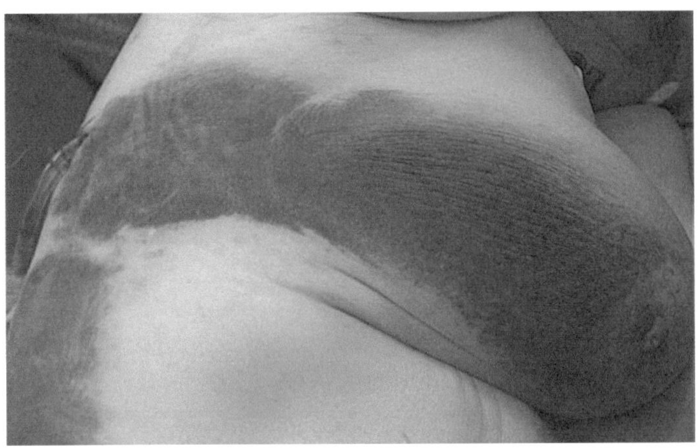

Chest wall hematoma 1

Injuries to the intercostal vessels as well as their subsequent branches or to the *A. thoracica lateralis* may lead to excessive bleeding requiring surgery.

Injuries to the vasculature are usually evident during the procedure. Venous injuries may remain undetected due to compression by the chest tube until the drain is removed [44]. Bleeding into the chest cavity with resultant anemia and hemothorax can lead to significant morbidity and mortality.

Late complications are seen even after several years such as arteriovenous fistulas that require surgery or embolization [19].

When choosing the subaxillary "safe triangle", potential injuries to the latissimus dorsi muscle and the vessel/nerve bundle can be avoided. Damages to these structures can cause hematomas and/or functional limitations like *scapula alata* [17].

More anterior localization can lead to issues of the breast including mastitis, pain, and complications with breast implants (i.e. a silicone-leak or silicothorax if disrupted) [41].

Soft tissue infections (see drain fixation) include those caused by pathogenic "routine germs" such a Staph. aureus

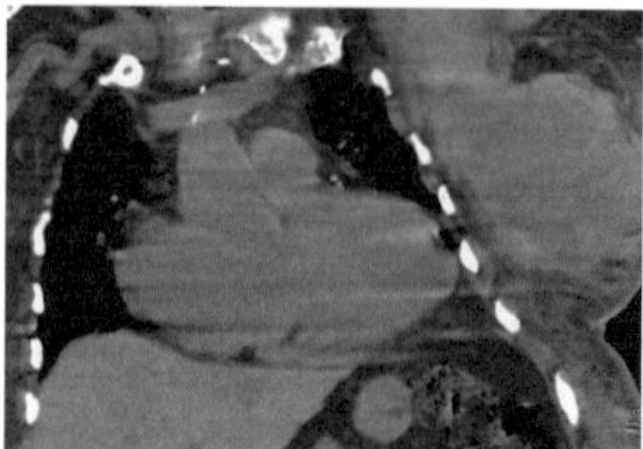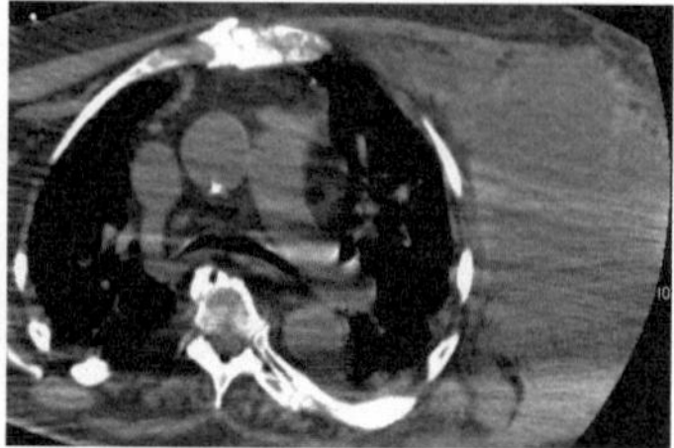

Chest wall haematoma 2+3

up to very serious cases of necrotizing fasciits [9, 21]. The latter might be difficult to differentiate in the presence of subcutaneous emphysema. Once recognized this is a surgical emergency requiring immediate intervention and antibiotic therapy. "Simple" wound infections can usually be cured with local treatment and may disappear after drain removal without systemic therapy. Erosion of ribs with consecutive osteomyelitis is very rare.

Sterile and an atraumatic surgical technique are fundamental principles for prevention of infection. There is no clear evidence to support prophylactic periinterventional administration of antibiotics. These antibiotics are mainly used in the emergency setting especially with penetrating chest trauma.

Damage to lung parenchyma can be caused by a soft tissue infection that is propagated along the chest tube. The chest tube can act as a "guardrail" from the extrathoracic space into the chest cavity. Insufficient evacuation of traumatic hemothoraces can lead to the development of blood clots and a restrictive pulmonary rind [12, 26]. In those patients, early thoracoscopic intervention to prevent empyema is recommended.

7.4.2   Damage of Lung Parenchyma

The organ most frequently injured during the insertion of a chest drain is the lung due to numerous reasons. The use of a chest drain with insufficient guidance along the inner

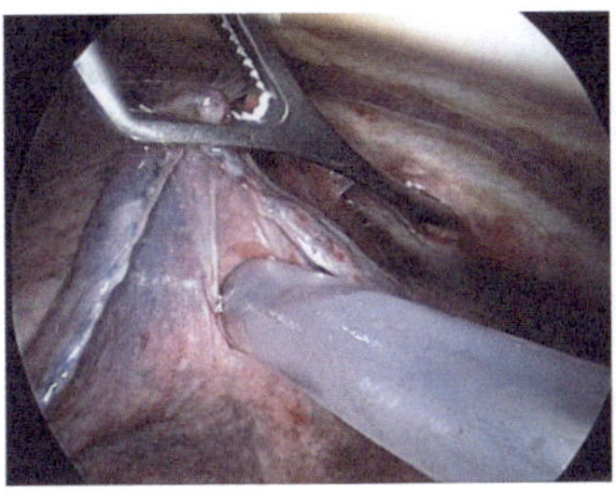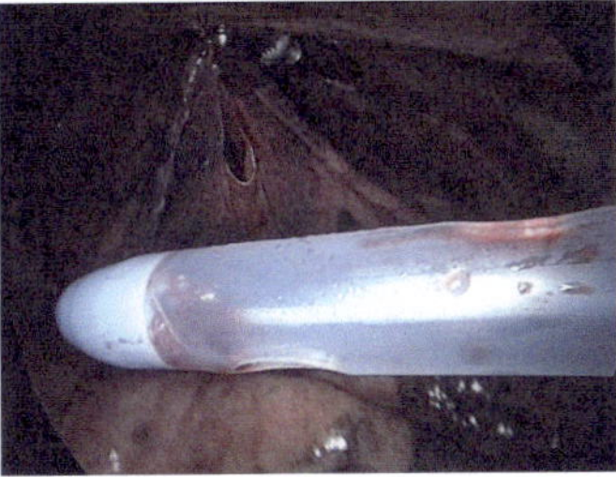

Injury of the lung parenchyma 1+2

convex surface of the chest wall can direct it in a perpendicular direction [34]. This can lead to injuries of the lung parenchyma as well as insufficient tube placement in the fissure.

Postinflammatory or postoperative adhesions are usually identified by sufficient preinterventional imaging (X-ray, CT scan) and taken into account when placing the drain.

In ventilated patients the lung does not develop atelectasis after opening of the parietal pleura and therefore the lung tissue does not fall away from the palpating finger. This can lead to parenchymal damage [13] which can be avoided by using short breaks in ventilation or apnea to insert the drain.

A cerebral air embolism can occur in ventilated patients after traumatic perforation of lung tissue or the intraparenchymal placement of a drain [5]. A lack of differential diagnostic considerations of this complication and the variable clinical symptoms may mask the real incidence of this complication.

A Broncopleural fistula may be an indication for chest drain insertion. To determine the correct diagnosis, CT scan, bronchoscopy, and bronchography may be used. Depending on the findings, treatment can be conservative after placement of a chest tube, endoscopic (endobronchial placement of valves, fibrin glue), or involve surgery.

Secondary parenchymal damage can be caused by insufficient fixation of the tube or an excessive application of suction [40].

Misinterpretation of bullous emphysema as a pneumothorax is a special instance where iatrogenic damage of lung parenchyma can be caused by placing a drain into the bulla. If there is any diagnostic doubt of disease, advanced imaging with a CT scan is mandatory.

Misinterpretation of bullous emphysema as a pneumothorax can lead to a prolonged air leak that frequently requires surgical intervention. A CT scan is mandatory if there is any doubt concerning the correct diagnosis.

Often damage of lung parenchyma is not noticed initially and later detected when high flow and/or insufficient drainage is observed. To avoid (tension) pneumothorax or extensive subcutaneous emphysema, a new drain should be placed prior to the removal of the original tube. Additional treatment will be dictated by the clinical course and may include continued current therapy or surgical repair of the damaged parenchyma (i.e. by a thoracoscopic intervention).

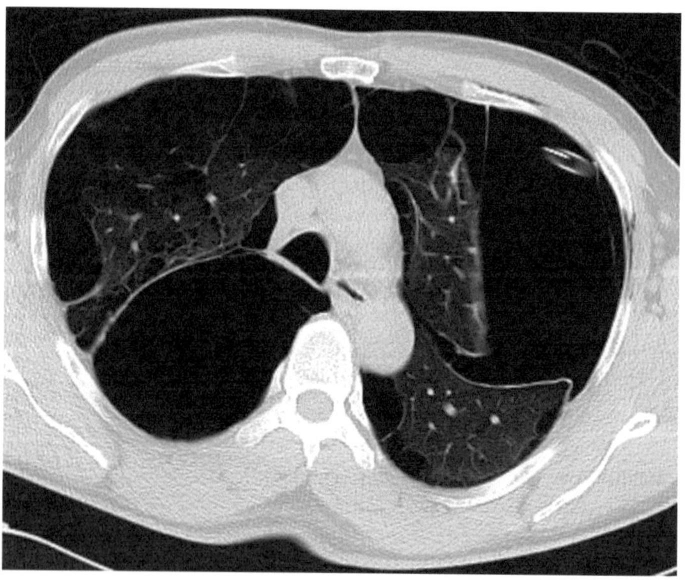

Injury of the lung parenchyma 3

7.4.3 Pleural Bleeding

When a malignant pleural effusion is caused by malignant pleural mesothelioma or other large malignant pleural tumors there is a potential bleeding risk. Development of a hemothorax that threatens the patient more than the initial effusion can occur. An ultrasound guided drain is recommended to avoid transtumoral placement. Bleeding caused by a chest tube in this situation can lead to an emergency thoracotomy and palliative pleurectomy or packing for hemostasis.

7.4.4 Heart and Blood Vessel Injuries

Previous operations (i.e. pneumonectomy) [30], trauma (flail chest caused by several rib fractures), chest deformity (kyphoscoliosis), hypertrophy of the heart [27], emergency

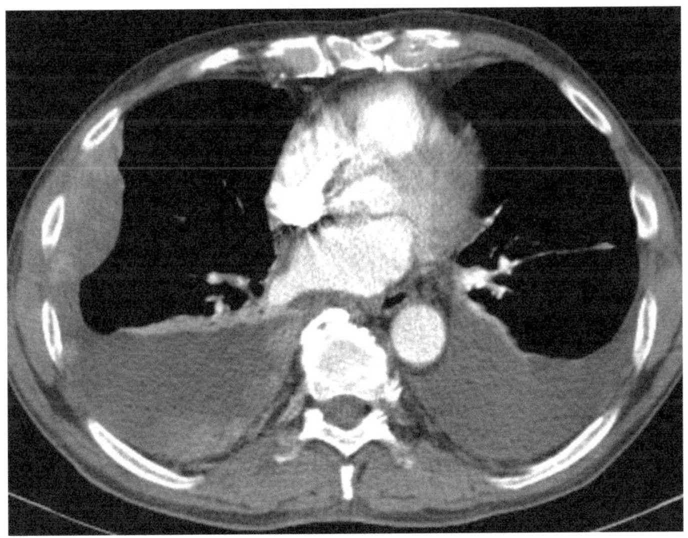

Effusion in pleural tumors

situations, and the use of trocar drains are predisposing factors for injury to the heart and great vessels. Immediate significant continuous and sometimes pulsatile bleeding in combination with hypotension should lead to the diagnosis. The immediate clamping of the drain left in situ may prevent fatal hemorrhage from occurring.

An immediate surgical intervention must follow [15, 28]. If the pulmonary artery is completely damaged beyond repair, a pneumonectomy will be the consequence. A conservative strategy of pulling back the chest drain sequentially day by day resulting in a clotting of the pulmonary artery has been described [48]. This is not recommended because of the hereby induced pulmonary embolism followed by cardiac stress and insecure control of coagulation.

7.4.5   Injuries of the Esophagus

Damage to the esophagus is infrequent and is usually due to mediastinal placement of the chest drain. These injuries include perforations and issues related to underlying esophageal pathologies. The finding of saliva or food particles in the chest tube or a newly detected air leak can raise the suspicion for such an injury. The treatment strategy will be determined by imaging (CT scan, contrast swallow, and esophagoscopy). Management may include surgery with primary suture repair of the defect with or without tissue coverage, stent implantation, or a purely conservative treatment including a chest drain.

7.4.6   Chylothorax

The Thoracic duct *(Ductus thoracic)* runs in a variable way along the esophagus and aorta. When the Thoracic duct is injured, the chest drainage may change to a milky fluid with a pathognomonic composition (triglyceride above 110 mg/dl) [32].

A parenteral diet limited to middle chain fatty acids usually stops the production of the chylus fluid. Other therapeutic options include thoracoscopic or open duct ligation, radiation of the mediastinum, and lymphografic embolization.

7.4.7 Mechanical Thoracic Irritation

Clinically relevant complications due to the drain can occur even when the chest tube is placed correctly in the pleural space.

In particular, the anatomy of children is such that the aorta, ventricles, and coronary arteries may be harmed due to hemodynamic relevant compression. Patient can also suffer from cardiogenic shock in a similar fashion which can be ameliorated by correct tube placement [22, 29, 47].

Complications including hematoma in the mediastinum or pericardum, erosions of the lung tissue, the esophagus and aorta have been described. When the clinical course is not straightforward, these potential complications have to be taken into account [2, 45, 53].

Drain related cardiac arrhythmias may challenge the physician's differential diagnostic abilities as medical treatment is not successful. Bradyarrhythmia and asystole can be caused by vagal nerve injury [55]. Tachyarrhythmia resistant to medical treatment that appear in a close context with the placement of a chest tube may be due to irritation of the pericardium and pressure on the ventricles. These problems are treated by removal of the chest drain [4, 7, 20].

When the tip of the chest tube places pressure on the apex of the chest cavity at the site of the sympathetic chain, a Horner's syndrome may occur resulting in the typical symptoms: miosis, ptosis, and anhidrosis. The severity and duration of symptoms is related to the location of the drain and latency until repositioning may occur [2].

Irritation of the phrenic nerve followed by diaphragmatic elevation is a very rare complication mainly seen in infants [37]. Respiratory limitation or a new radiological finding of Chilaiditi syndrome may be indirect clinical signs [42].

7.4.8   Injuries of Abdominal Organs

The apex of the diaphragm extends at the end of expiration up to the fifth intercostal space on the left side and to the fourth intercostal space on the right. To avoid injuries to the diaphragm and the intraabdominal organs, it is strongly recommended that a chest drain inserted under emergency conditions never be placed below the forth intercostal space. The forth intercostal space is located at the nipple in men and around the inframammary line in women.

At the end of expiration, the apex of the diaphragm extends up to the fifth intercostal space on the left side and to the fourth intercostal space on the right. To avoid injuries to the diaphragm and the intraabdominal organs, it is strongly recommended that when a chest drain is inserted under emergency conditions, it should never be placed below the fourth intercostal space.

There are many etiologies that can cause elevation of the diaphragm (i.e. Lesions of the phrenic nerve postoperatively or after trauma, ascites, pregnancy, etc.).

Diaphragmatic injuries due to chest drain insertion may lead to life threatening thoracic and/or intraabdominal bleeding which is initially asymptomatic. If a patient is clinically deteriorating after chest tube removal, one must consider tamponade as a possible etiology.

Damage to the stomach or bowel are increased in patients with an elevated diaphragm as well as when a trocar drain is used. One must consider traumatic rupture of the diaphragm in patients who have undergone trauma. Gastrothorax or enterothorax may present on a chest x-ray as a (tension) pneumothorax which could lead to inadequate management in a patient presenting with respiratory disorders or circulatory shock. Perforation of a hollow organ always needs surgical intervention.

The placement of a chest tube in the liver or spleen is a rare complication. Clinical symptoms can range from asymptomatic to acute life threatening bleeding requiring diagnostic confirmation and emergency procedures [1].

Treatment options should be chosen according to the degree of damage which can include drain removal and close observation, percutaneous interventions (i.e. hepatic embolization) [50] as well as (emergency) laparotomy to exclude further intraabdominal damage.

7.4.9   Re-expansion Edema

Reexpansion edema is a quite rare but potentially life threatening complication following reexpansion of the lung after relief of a pneumothorax or pleural effusion. Incidence is reported up to 20 %.

The pathophysiology is not clear. A combination of causes such as compression of lung tissue, mechanical forces, reexpansion, hypoxic liberation of radicals, and immunological processes are followed by an increased endothelial permeability. This leads to damaged capillary leakage in alveoli with consecutive exudation.

Risk factors include age over 40, more than 30 % lung tissue compression, tension pneumothorax, 3+ days of compression more than three days, and a fast reexpansion with high negative pressure. When a effusion is relieved with the assistance of pleural monitoring with a pressure set point less negative than -20 cm H_2O there is a significant risk reduction. Consensus guidelines recommend a fractional relief with no more than 1500 ml removed at one time [18, 33].

Clinical symptoms include cough, dyspnea, chest pain, tachycardia, and hypoxia as well as a decreased transparency on the x-ray within 1–2 h after the intervention.

Treatment should include closely monitoring, administration of oxygen, supine positioning with the affected side up, diuretic therapy, and possibly mechanical ventilation or hemodynamic supportive medication. Administration of NSAR and glucocorticoids is established but is not evidence based [10, 14].

When reexpansion edema occurs, it typically appears within 1–2 h after reexpansion of the lung. Risk factors for

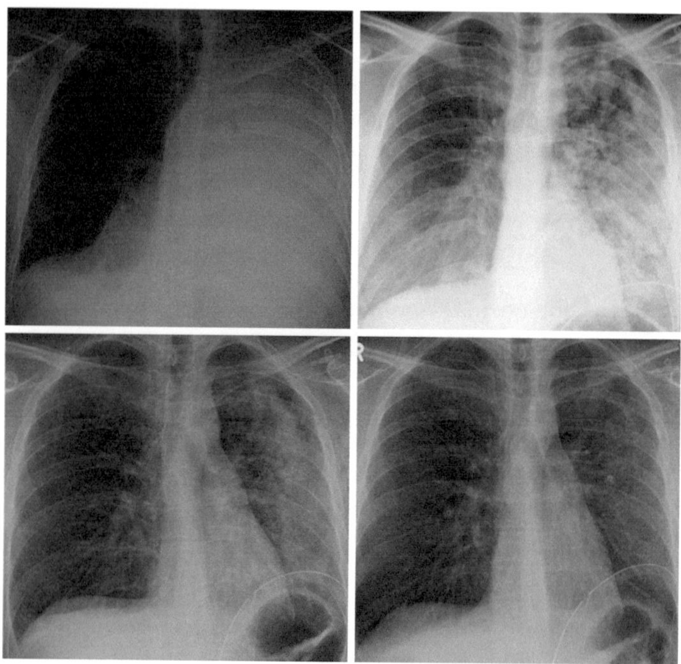

Re-expansion edema

the development of reexpansion edema include age <40 years, more than 30 % of compressed lung, tension pneumothorax, compression of the lung more than three days, and fast decompression.

7.5   Control of Findings

A chest xray and/or ultrasound in recommended to help monitor anatomical reasons for any symptoms and the clinical course (with or without complication) related to an intervention. If findings are not clear, a CT scan should be added to detect if there has been insufficient intervention, complications, or residual findings that need treatment ([6, 31, 39]).

Literature: Complications

1. Bae JM. Life threatening hemoperitoneum and liver injury as a result of chest tube thoracostomy. Clin Med Insights. Case reports 2001;8:15–7. PMC [article] PMCID: PMC4345926, PMID: 25780345. doi:10.4137/CCRep.S23139.
2. Baird R, Al-Balushi Z, Wackett J, Bouchard S. Iatrogenic Horner syndrome after tube thoracostomy. J Pediatr Surg. 2009;44(10):2012–4. doi:10.1016/j.jpedsurg.2009.05.022. PubMed [citation] PMID: 19853764.
3. Ball CG, Lord J, Laupland KB, Gmora S, Mulloy RH, Ng AK, Schieman C, Kirkpatrick AW. Chest tube complications: how well are we training our residents? Can J Surg. 2007;50(6):450–8. PubMed [citation] PMID: 18053373, PMCID: PMC2386217.
4. Barak M, Iaroshevski D, Ziser A. Rapid atrial fibrillation following tube thoracostomy insertion. Eur J Cardiothorac Surg. 2003;24(3):461–2. PubMed [citation] PMID: 12965324.
5. Brownlow HA, Edibam C. Systemic air embolism after intercostal chest drain insertion and positive pressure ventilation in chest trauma. Anaesth Intensive Care. 2002;30(5):660–4. PubMed [citation] PMID: 12413269.
6. Cameron EW, Mirvis SE, Shanmuganathan K, White CS, Miller BH. Computed tomography of malpositioned thoracostomy drains: a pictorial essay. Clin Radiol. 1997;52(3):187–93. Review. PubMed [citation] PMID: 9091252.
7. Cardozo S, Belgrave K. A shocking complication of a pneumothorax: chest tube-induced arrhythmias and review of the literature. Case Rep Cardiol. 2014;2014:681572. doi:10.1155/2014/681572. Epub 2014 Jul 24. PubMed [citation] PMID: 25147742, PMCID: PMC4131458.
8. Chan L, Reilly KM, Henderson C, Kahn F, Salluzzo RF. Complication rates of tube thoracostomy. Am J Emerg Med. 1997;15(4):368–70. PubMed [citation] PMID: 9217527.
9. Chen YM, Wu MF, Lee PY, Su WJ, Perng RP. Necrotizing fasciitis: is it a fatal complication of tube thoracostomy? Report of three cases. Respir Med. 1992;86(3):249–51. No abstract available. PubMed [citation] PMID: 1620913.
10. Cho SR, Lee JS, Kim MS. New treatment method for reexpansion pulmonary edema: differential lung ventilation. Ann Thorac Surg. 2005;80(5):1933–4. PubMed [citation] PMID: 16242493.

11. Da Rocha RP, Vengjer A, Blanco A, de Carvalho PT, Mongon ML, Fernandes GJ. Size of the collateral intercostal artery in adults: anatomical considerations in relation to thoracocentesis and thoracoscopy. Surg Radiol Anat. 2002;24(1):23–6. PubMed [citation] PMID: 12197006.

12. DuBose J, Inaba K, Okoye O, Demetriades D, Scalea T, O'Connor J, Menaker J, Morales C, Shiflett T, Brown C, Copwood B, AAST Retained Hemothorax Study Group. Development of posttraumatic empyema in patients with retained hemothorax: results of a prospective, observational AAST study. J Trauma Acute Care Surg. 2012;73(3):752–7. PubMed [citation] PMID: 22929504.

13. Etoch SW, Bar-Natan MF, Miller FB, Richardson JD. Tube thoracostomy. Factors related to complications. Arch Surg. 1995;130(5):521–5; discussion 525–6. PubMed [citation] PMID: 7748091.

14. Feller-Kopman D, Berkowitz D, Boiselle P, Ernst A. Large-volume thoracentesis and the risk of reexpansion pulmonary edema. Ann Thorac Surg. 2007;84(5):1656–61. PubMed [citation] PMID: 17954079.

15. Goltz JP, Gorski A, Böhler J, Kickuth R, Hahn D, Ritter CO. Iatrogenic perforation of the left heart during placement of a chest drain. Diagn Interv Radiol. 2011;17(3):229–31. doi:10.4261/1305-3825.DIR.3131-09.0. Epub 2010 Aug 3. PubMed [citation] PMID: 20683819.

16. Harris A, O'Driscoll BR, Turkington PM. Survey of major complications of intercostal chest drain insertion in the UK. Postgrad Med J. 2010;86(1012):68–72. doi:10.1136/pgmj.2009.087759. PubMed [citation] PMID: 20145053.

17. Hassan WU, Keaney NP. Winging of the scapula: an unusual complication of chest tube placement. J Accid Emerg Med. 1995;12(2):156–7. PubMed [citation] PMID: 7582419, PMCID: PMC1342561.

18. Havelock T, Teoh R, Laws D, Gleeson F, BTS Pleural Disease Guideline Group. Pleural procedures and thoracic ultrasound: British Thoracic Society Pleural Disease Guideline 2010. Thorax. 2010;65(Suppl 2):ii61–76. doi:10.1136/thx.2010.137026. No abstract available. PubMed [citation] PMID: 20696688.

19. Heifetz SA, Zeichner MB, Minkowitz S. Sudden death from ruptured intercostal artery aneurysm. A late complication of thoracotomy. Arch Surg. 1975;110(10):1253–4. No abstract available. PubMed [citation] PMID: 1191.

20. Hibbert B, Lim TW, Hibbert R, Green M, Gollob MH, Davis DR. Ventricular tachycardia following tube thoracotomy. Europace. 2010;12(10):1504–6. doi:10.1093/europace/euq172. Epub 2010 Jun 4. PubMed [citation] PMID: 20525725.
21. Hsu SP, Wang HC, Huang IT, Chu KA, Chang HC. Tube thoracostomy-related necrotizing fasciitis: a case report. Kaohsiung J Med Sci. 2006;22(12):636–40. PubMed [citation] PMID: 17116626.
22. Iaci G, Castiglioni A, Fumero A, Carlino M, Margonato A, Alfieri O. Resolution of an acute cardiac ischemia after the removal of a surgical drain in mitral and tricuspid valve repair. Ann Thorac Surg. 2011;91(6):e94. doi:10.1016/j.athoracsur.2011.03.018. No abstract available. PubMed [citation] PMID: 21619958.
23. Jeon EY, Cho YK, Yoon DY, Seo YL, Lim KJ, Yun EJ. Angiographic analysis of the lateral intercostal artery perforator of the posterior intercostal artery: anatomic variation and clinical significance. Diagn Interv Radiol. 2015;21(5):415–8. PMC [article] PMCID: PMC4557326, PMID: 26268302. doi:10.5152/dir.2015.15096.
24. John M, Razi S, Sainathan S, Stavropoulos C. Is the trocar technique for tube thoracostomy safe in the current era? Interact Cardiovasc Thorac Surg. 2014;19(1):125–8. doi:10.1093/icvts/ivu071. Epub 2014 Mar 19. Review. PubMed [citation] PMID: 24648468.
25. Jones PM, Hewer RD, Wolfenden HD, Thomas PS. Subcutaneous emphysema associated with chest tube drainage. Respirology. 2001;6(2):87–9. PubMed [citation] PMID: 11422886.
26. Karmy-Jones R, Holevar M, Sullivan RJ, Fleisig A, Jurkovich GJ. Residual hemothorax after chest tube placement correlates with increased risk of empyema following traumatic injury. Can Respir J. 2008;15(5):255–8. PubMed [citation] PMID: 18716687, PMCID: PMC2679547.
27. Kerger H, Blaettner T, Froehlich C, Ernst J, Frietsch T, Isselhorst C, Nguyen AK, Volz A, Fiedler F, Genzwuerker HV. Perforation of the left atrium by a chest tube in a patient with cardiomegaly: management of a rare, but life-threatening complication. Resuscitation. 2007;74(1):178–82. Epub 2007 Feb 14. PubMed [citation] PMID: 17303305.
28. Kim D, Lim SH, Seo PW. Iatrogenic perforation of the left ventricle during insertion of a chest drain. Korean J Thorac Cardiovasc Surg. 2013;46(3):223–5. doi:10.5090/kjtcs.2013.46.3.223. Epub 2013 Jun 5. PubMed [citation] PMID: 23772413, PMCID: PMC3680611.

29. Kollef MH, Dothager DW. Reversible cardiogenic shock due to chest tube compression of the right ventricle. Chest. 1991;99(4):976–80. PubMed [citation] PMID: 2009805.
30. Kopec SE, Conlan AA, Irwin RS. Perforation of the right ventricle: a complication of blind placement of a chest tube into the postpneumonectomy space. Chest. 1998;114(4):1213–5. PubMed [citation] PMID: 9792599.
31. Landay M, Oliver Q, Estrera A, Friese R, Boonswang N, DiMaio JM. Lung penetration by thoracostomy tubes: imaging findings on CT. J Thorac Imaging. 2006;21(3):197–204.
32. Limsukon A, Yick D, Kamangar N. Chylothorax: a rare complication of tube thoracostomy. J Emerg Med. 2011;40(3):280–2. doi:10.1016/j.jemermed.2007.12.023. Epub 2008 Aug 30. PubMed [citation] PMID: 18757158.
33. Maskell NA, Butland RJ, Pleural Diseases Group, Standards of Care Committee, British Thoracic Society. BTS guidelines for the investigation of a unilateral pleural effusion in adults. Thorax. 2003;58 Suppl 2:ii8–17. No abstract available. PubMed [citation] PMID: 12728146, PMCID: PMC1766019.
34. Maybauer MO, Geisser W, Wolff H, Maybauer DM. Incidence and outcome of tube thoracostomy positioning in trauma patients. Prehosp Emerg Care. 2012;16(2):237–41. doi:10.3109/10903127.2011.615975. Epub 2011 Oct 3. PubMed [citation] PMID: 21967410.
35. Millikan JS, Moore EE, Steiner E, Aragon GE, Van Way CW 3rd. Complications of tube thoracostomy for acute trauma. Am J Surg. 1980;140(6):738–41. PubMed [citation] PMID: 7457693.
36. Muthuswamy P, Samuel J, Mizock B, Dunne P. Recurrent massive bleeding from an intercostal artery aneurysm through an empyema chest tube. Chest. 1993;104(2):637–9. PubMed [citation] PMID: 8339668.
37. Nahum E, Ben-Ari J, Schonfeld T, Horev G (2001) Acute diaphragmatic paralysis caused by chest-tube trauma to phrenic nerve. Pediatr Radiol 31:444–6; PMID: 11436893.
38. Paul AO, Kirchhoff C, Kay MV, Hiebl A, Koerner M, Braunstein VA, Mutschler W, Kanz KG. Malfunction of a Heimlich flutter valve causing tension pneumothorax: case report of a rare complication. Patient Saf Surg. 2010;4(1):8. doi:10.1186/1754-9493-4-8. PubMed [citation] PMID: 20565768, PMCID: PMC2901307.
39. Remérand F, Luce V, Badachi Y, Lu Q, Bouhemad B, Rouby JJ. Incidence of chest tube malposition in the critically ill: a prospective computed tomography study. Anesthesiology. 2007;106(6):1112–9. PubMed [citation] PMID: 17525585.

40. Resnick DK. Delayed pulmonary perforation. A rare complication of tube thoracostomy. Chest. 1993;103(1):311–3. PubMed [citation] PMID: 8417916.
41. Rice DC, Agasthian T, Clay RP, Deschamps C. Silicone thorax: a complication of tube thoracostomy in the presence of mammary implants. Ann Thorac Surg. 1995;60(5):1417–9. Review. PubMed [citation] PMID: 8526644.
42. Salon JE. Reversible diaphragmatic eventration following chest tube thoracostomy. Ann Emerg Med. 1995;25(4):556–8. Review. PubMed [citation] PMID: 7710170.
43. Schmidt U, Stalp M, Gerich T, Blauth M, Maull KI, Tscherne H. Chest tube decompression of blunt chest injuries by physicians in the field: effectiveness and complications. J Trauma. 1998;44(1):98–101. PubMed [citation] PMID: 9464755.
44. Seki M, Yoda S. Unexpected massive hemorrhage following the removal of a pleural drainage tube. Intern Med. 2015;54(8):953–4. doi:10.2169/internalmedicine.54.3719. Epub 2015 Apr 15. PubMed [citation] PMID: 25876579.
45. Shapira OM, Aldea GS, Kupferschmid J, Shemin RJ. Delayed perforation of the esophagus by a closed thoracostomy tube. Chest. 1993;104(6):1897–8. PubMed [citation] PMID: 8252980.
46. Shojaee S, Argento AC. Ultrasound-guided pleural access. Semin Respir Crit Care Med. 2014;35(6):693–705. doi:10.1055/s-0034-1395794. Epub 2014 Dec 2. Review. PubMed [citation] PMID: 25463160.
47. Sulimovic S, Noyez L. Postoperative myocardial ischemia caused by compression of a coronary artery by chest tube. J Cardiovasc Surg (Torino). 2006;47(3):371–2. No abstract available. PubMed [citation] PMID: 16760877.
48. Sundaramurthy SR, Moshinsky RA, Smith JA. Non-operative management of tube thoracostomy induced pulmonary artery injury. Interact Cardiovasc Thorac Surg. 2009;9(4):759–60. doi:10.1510/icvts.2009.209262. Epub 2009 Jul 31. PubMed [citation] PMID: 19648149.
49. Svedjeholm R, Håkanson E. Postoperative myocardial ischemia caused by chest tube compression of vein graft. Ann Thorac Surg. 1997;64(6):1806–8. PubMed [citation] PMID: 9436578.
50. Tait P, Waheed U, Bell S. Successful removal of malpositioned chest drain within the liver by embolization of the transhepatic track. Cardiovasc Intervent Radiol. 2009;32(4):825–7. doi:10.1007/s00270-008-9461-y. Epub 2008 Oct 30. PubMed [citation] PMID: 18972157.

51. Waydhas C, Sauerland S. Pre-hospital pleural decompression and chest tube placement after blunt trauma: a systematic review. Resuscitation. 2007;72(1):11–25. Epub 2006 Nov 22. Review. PubMed [citation] PMID: 17118508.
52. Wraight WM, Tweedie DJ, Parkin IG. Neurovascular anatomy and variation in the fourth, fifth, and sixth intercostal spaces in the mid-axillary line: a cadaveric study in respect of chest drain insertion. Clin Anat. 2005;18(5):346–9. PubMed [citation] PMID: 15971216.
53. Yen CC, Yang YS, Liu KY. Aortic perforation caused by friction of a chest tube after coronary artery bypass surgery. Heart Surg Forum. 2010;13(3):E159–60. doi:10.1532/HSF98.20091165. PubMed [citation] PMID: 20534415.
54. Yoneyama H, Arahata M, Temaru R, Ishizaka S, Minami S. Evaluation of the risk of intercostal artery laceration during thoracentesis in elderly patients by using 3D-CT angiography. Intern Med. 2010;49(4):289–92. Epub 2010 Feb 15. PubMed [citation] PMID: 20154433.
55. Ward EW, Hughes TE (1994) Sudden death following chest tube insertion: and unusual case pf vagus nerve irritation. J Trauma 36:258–259.

Chapter 8
Care of Patients Having a Chest Drain

Fabian Graeb

8.1   Monitoring and Management of Chest Drains

All aspects of the chest drain and system as well as the patient's condition need to be monitored very closely. The information obtained by the nursing staff is important and is in turn the basis for therapeutic decisions. Therefore the information obtained has to be integrated into daily workflow. Particular details during each patient contact include:

- How does the patient feel and is there any concern over his/her condition?
- Does the chest drain system work in the correct manner? Are the physician's requirements fulfilled?
- Are the settings of the chest drainage system correct?
- How much air leak and fluid production has there been in past 24 h and how does it compare to previous days?
- Does the data make sense?
- Are there sudden changes which cannot be explained that need to be investigated?

F. Graeb
Karl-Olga-Krankenhaus ICU
Hackstraße 61, 70190 Stuttgart, Germany
e-mail: Fabian.Graeb@googlemail.com

© Springer International Publishing Switzerland 2017
T. Kiefer (ed.), *Chest Drains in Daily Clinical Practice*,
DOI 10.1007/978-3-319-32339-8_8

When concerning changes or complications occur the physician in charge has to be informed immediately and documented appropriately.

8.1.1 Monitoring of the Chest Drain System

Detailed knowledge concerning the construction and operation of the chest drain system are mandatory. Without this knowledge, the correct function of the system cannot be guaranteed. This lack of knowledge also could lead to serious complications if trouble shooting or malfunction occurs. Training has to be offered to the nursing staff as a routine procedure making sure to include any new staff members or part time employees. Regardless which system is in use, the following issues have to be checked:

- Is the negative pressure set on the system correct? In analogous systems where a manometer sets the pressure, the pressure may have been inadvertently changed and needs correction. In addition there may be variations as there is an air leak. In the case of a bigger air leak, the oscillation of the manometer's needles can be detected. One must also check that the system is connected to the suction source.
- In electronic systems the set pressure always has to be checked and compared with the individual requirements for that patient. An unintended change is less likely with the electronic system.
- Is the system assembled in the proper way?
- Is the system properly connected with the chest drain? In particular when using analogous systems it might take some time before this fault is detected with the consequence of a pneumothorax. This could lead to a pleural infection if the drain is disconnected over a longer time period.
- With an analogue system: Is there a sufficient amount of water in the corresponding compartments of the system? The water levels must be monitored as some of the water that was initially filled may evaporate, especially when there is a bigger air leak.

8.1.2   Parameters to Be Noticed During Therapy

The most important parameters that guide therapeutic decision making during chest drain therapy (besides a chest xray) are the air leak and fluid production. There is a huge variety in what is expected for these two parameters depending on the underlying disease, the procedure done, and the individual therapeutic course.

8.1.2.1   Pleural Fluid Production

When examining the fluid produced assess:

- Fluid amount

  - look, color, viscosity
  - smell
  - sudden changes (i.e. Unexpected low fluid production)

If there are sudden changes concerning the look and the amount of fluid output, the physician in charge has to be informed immediately and the fluid analyzed (Table 8.1). The drain may be clogged if there is a sudden significant decrease

TABLE 8.1 Kinds of pleural effusions

Description of the fluid	Explanation and possible causes
Serous, slightly yellow	Normal pleural fluid
Purulent, murky	
Sanguineous	Hemothorax: injury of a blood vessel (i.e. intercostal vessel)
White or milky (rare)	Chylus: due to injury of the ductus thoracic
Black (very rare)	Distinct fungal infection, melanoma, pancreatopleural fistula
Green/brown, high viscosity, sour smell (very rare)	Esophagopleural fistula

Source: Bölükbas et al. [1], Eggeling [6], Saraya et al. [13], and Sziklavari et al. [15]

in the fluid production and the system needs to be checked. Using an analogue system, a so-called "swing test" can be helpful: There needs to be some fluid in the tubing to be able to lock the tubing. The patient is asked to take a couple of deep breathes. If the fluid in the tubing swings, this is a strong hint that the tubing is at least partly open. If not, the tubing is likely clogged. It is not a sign that gives 100 % significance. Electronic systems have a software related feature that demonstrates the breath related differences in pressure.

The fluid output threshold for chest drain removal differs from hospital to hospital. In general the underlying disease and the quality of the fluid have to be taken in account (i.e. empyema drains are removed when fluid cultures are negative). Chest tubes can be safely removed with daily fluid output of up to 450 ml as long as the fluid is non suspicious [2, 3, 15].

If there is any doubt about the quality of the pleural fluid then analysis should be done. Most drainage systems have a sample port with a membrane either in the tubing or the collection chamber. The protocol for taking a sample is more or less the same as taking a sample from a urinary catheter: The sample port is disinfected and then sterilely sampled with a syringe after waiting 30 seconds. This is then sent to the lab. If the fluid is suspicious for an empyema then a corresponding microbiological analysis should be done. Milky fluid suspicious for a chylothorax should be sent for a triglyceride level as well as a triglyceride level in the patient's blood [1].

8.1.2.2   Air Leak

An "air leak" is due to leakage from the lung parenchyma or a bronchus. An air leak becomes visible as bubbling in the water seal chamber in an analogue system or as a precise and objective numeric number when using an electronic system. The appearance and clinical course of such an air leak has to be watched and documented. According to experience, an air leak may change over time with quite a wide range. Sometimes the difference is due to patient positioning (i.e. bigger in an upright position compared to when lying supine). Sudden changes such as the appearance of a new air leak or sudden cessation of a leak must be reported to the physician in charge immediately. In the latter case, the system and the tube should be checked regarding patency. As the appearance or persistence of an air leak is a contraindication to drain removal one must ensure that the air leak is "real". Air leaks can also be due to issues with the tubing and/or the system and these must be ruled out. The same approach of checking the tubing and system should be undertaken when a huge, persisting air leak is observed (Table 8.2).

8.1.3   *Management of Chest Drain Systems*

The chest drain system should be positioned in such a way that all relevant components (collection chamber, manometer or water seal) can be checked easily during each contact with the patient. Furthermore an unintended overthrow of the system must be avoided. Most systems must be placed underneath the chest as this is the only way to guarantee unhampered drainage. Electronic systems with double lumen technique can be positioned anywhere.

8.1.3.1   Siphon

To avoid the so called siphon effect, the tubing has to be arranged in a way that a loop is not created. As fluid accumulates in this loop the negative pressure set at the manometer or the pressure chamber is reduced by the height of the fluid column (i.e. the pressure is set at -20 cm of water, the fluid column in the siphon is 20 cm as well and therefore no negative pressure is applied to the pleural cavity). Working with a water seal without a suction source, a siphon of 20 cm will generate a negative pressure of -20 cm of water in the pleural space. Therefore the tubing must always be placed in a way to avoid a siphon. Whenever a siphon filled with fluid is noticed, the fluid has to be directed towards the system's collection chamber.

This situation appears only can occur when using an analogue system without the possibility of monitoring the pressure next to the patient. If one is using an electronic system with double lumen tubing, the siphon effect does not exist [10].

Chest drains should never be clamped for patient transport.

8.1.3.2   Mobilization and Transport

Patient's mobilization and the need for transport can lead to some practical problems when a drainage system is in use. Mobilization limitation may be due to the drainage system needing to be connected to a suction source. When the patient needs to leave the bed to be transported to another location (i.e. the radiological department) the analogue system usually has to be disconnected from the wall suction source. Most commonly wall suction is the common way of generating negative pressure when using these analogue systems. One must remember that the drain should never be clamped because the patient is being moved! Clamping the drain is widely done, but has no advantages. Doing so can be life threatening as a tension pneumothorax can occur as air from an air leak can no longer be evacuated from the chest cavity. In a patient with an air leak, disconnection from suction can lead to lung collapse. Usually this problem is easily solved by reconnecting the system to suction. Clamping for a very short time only should only be done when needed for canister and/or tubing changing under close observation.

A chest drain cannot be an obstacle for patient mobilization!

In general, the following considerations should be taken into account when mobilizing a patient:

- The patient has to have adequate pain control. Moving chest drains can cause significant pain due to irritation of the corresponding intercostal nerve [12]. Routine pain assessment using a numeric ranking scale (NRS) in conjunction with appropriate analgesic medications is a neccessity.

- Some chest drain systems have long tubing that can act as a tripping hazard. Patients must be supported and well educated to avoid an accident.
- When it is necessary to obtain negative pressure during mobilization and/or transport the chest drain system has to be connected to a mobile suction source. In general all analogue systems can be hooked up with an electronic driven suction source.
- If oxygen or walking assistance devise are needed, they should be made available for use.
- When the patient is being mobilized for the first time after surgery or chest drain insertion, nursing staff should explain the process of moving with the apparatus attached. There should be adequate assistance provided to ensure mobilization is safe and optimized.
- The patient needs to know to immediately call for help if there is a change in condition such as dyspnea or if the chest drain system gets disconnected.

8.1.3.3 Changing the System and Securing Connections

Partial or complete change of the chest drain system is indicated when the collection canister is full or the system is damaged. The system needs to be reassembled according to the instructions for use. The water seal chamber and suction chamber are filled with water if a wet system is used. The tubing is clamped for a short time period so that the old system or full canister can be replaced. One must ensure the most hygienic exchange possible because contamination of the connection site must be avoided.

It is common practice to "secure" the connection site with plaster, tape, or cable ties in order to prevent any disconnection of the tubing. The use of plaster is not recommended as one cannot see underneath the plaster if a disconnection occurs and its use also hinders tubing changes. The latter is also true when using cable ties as the tie can only be removed

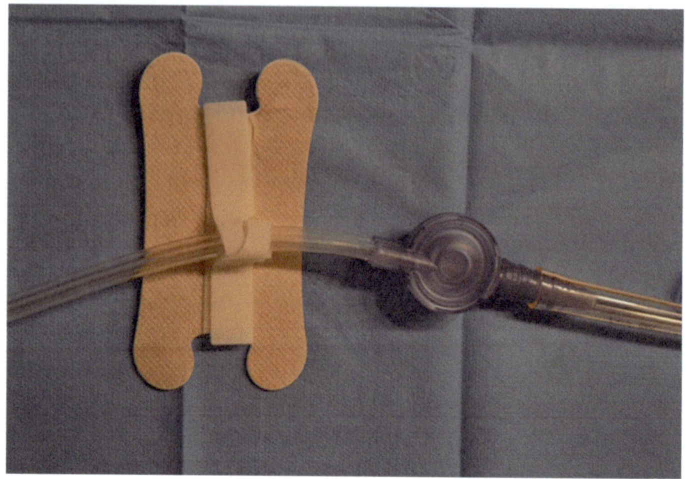

FIGURE 8.1 Example of a fixing system for chest drains

with a special tool that can damage the tubing during the process. If the patient steps on the tubing unintentionally, securing with a cable tie prevent disconnection but has the possibility to tear out the chest tube. As one can imagine, this would cause more problems than disconnected tubing and therefore cable ties are not recommended.

The use of special plaster loops to secure the tubing does make more sense. There are commercial systems available for fixation of chest tubes such as Secutape® (Fig. 8.1) or Tubimed® to secure the chest tube distally to the drainage system. These securing systems have a substrate fixed on the skin, a little loop for fixation of the tube glued around the tube, and are fixed on the substrate with a hook and pile fastener. These systems help to prevent disconnection without increasing the risk of an unintentional removal of the chest tube.

8.1.3.4   Stripping and Milking

"Milking" describes pressing on a chest tube to move intraluminal fluid or debris. Stripping is a maneuver that uses a special instrument (a kind of a clamp with rolls) to create massive negative pressure in the tubing, started next to the patient and then stripping towards the canister. For a long time this practice was widely used in many centers in a prophylactic manner to prevent the tubing from clogging. In doing so, a negative pressure of up to −400 cm of water could be generated. Several studies done in cardiac surgery patients have shown that there is no reduction of clogging by prophylactic milking of chest drains when stripping is used. The amount of fluid per day was increased which resulted in longer drainage times. Injuries to the pleura and lung could neither be detected nor excluded. Prophylactic milking and stripping is truly obsolete because of their ineffectiveness. If there is a strong suspicion of a clogged chest tube (sudden cessation of an air leak, fluid production stopped abruptly, visible clot), stripping or milking is then indicated [4, 9].

8.1.3.5   Leakage Test

Every drainage system has the potential for leakage due to improper use, damage, or failures during the manufacturing process (rare). Two situations are highly suspicious regarding the presence of a leakage within the system:

- The presence of an air leak that is not consistent with the history of the patient, which is new, persisting, and or stable in quantity
- The system is not able to create a negative pressure

Regardless which kind of system is used, the tightness can be efficiently and easily checked. First the tubing is clamped for a short time adjacent skin incision on the patient. If the leakage disappears and negative pressure is generated, the system and its connections are tight. This means that the "problem" is related to the patient or at least proximally to the clamp. If the leakage persists with clamping, the system or parts distal to the clamp have to be changed.

As a matter of principle, a test checking the tightness of the system should always be done before it is connected to the patient. To attain appropriate tightness, all components of the system have to be assembled properly. Whenever a component has to be connected with a screwing action or by putting on a cap, the probability for error that could cause a leak is increased. These potential points of failure have to be checked before every use. If the system does not generate negative pressure the suction source must be checked as well.

If there is no failure detected in the system, the skin incision has to be checked. The tube may have slipped out so far that air is sucked in by one of the tubes holes or the skin incision is too wide which allows air to be sucked in. To check the possibility of air being sucked in through the skin incision, a sterile fluid can be sprayed around the tube to see if it is sucked in. The problem may be solved if a stitch is placed to better reapproximate the incision around the tube. If failures of the system and the incision are ruled out, more severe causes of an air leak such as a bronchopleural fistula must be considered [11].

8.1.3.6   Trouble Shooting: Quick Overview

TABLE 8.2 Overview of possible problems, causes and solutions

Problem	Potential causes	Trouble shooting
Sudden appearance of a large air leak	Disconnection, Leakage in the system, New parenchymal damage, bronchial stump insufficiency	Check connection, if necessary reconnect tubing Check tightness of the system: clamp tubing next to the patient, if air leak persists >> change system Check skin incision: is the incision too wide? Is air being sucked in from outside? Has the drain slipped out?
Cessation of air leak and/or fluid production abruptly	Drain is clogged	Check tubing for clogging Milk or strip the tube if needed

(continued)

TABLE 8.2 (continued)

Problem	Potential causes	Trouble shooting
Dyspnea	Drain is clogged, No suction, Pneumonia, if shortly after drain insertion consider reexpansion edema (rare)	Check suction source, if necessary hook up a suction source If necessary check the system for a leak if no negative pressure is generated Check tubing concerning clamping, if necessary take off the clamp Check tubing for clogging, if necessary milk or strip tube If no or minimal improvement: call the physician in charge Severe dyspnea: always call the physician in charge Signs of pneumonia: fever, tachycardia, tachypnea: always call the physician in charge
Face and neck swelling	Subcutaneous emphysema due to a clogged chest tube or other reasons for insufficient therapy (i.e. malposition of the chest tube	Check for clogging, leakage, assess the skin incision and position of the drain, and set pressure Inform the physician in charge
Severe pain	Pain related to the chest tube, Pneumothorax	Check function of the drain and system (set pressure, patency) Drug administration If necessary adjust pain medication Discuss with the physician and physiotherapist

(continued)

TABLE 8.2 (continued)

Problem	Potential causes	Trouble shooting
Extreme increase in output (also Table 8.1)	According to clinical situation: Cardiac causes? Bleeding? Chylothorax? Infection?	Precise observation and documentation: amount, appearance, color, smell Inform physician in charge If necessary take a sample
Dressing saturation	Skin incision too big, infection of skin incision	Check skin incision, if necessary inform physician in charge

8.2   Monitoring and Support of the Patient

The patients treated with chest drains are a very heterogeneous group of people regarding age, underlying disease, and general physical condition. Nevertheless, any patient who has a chest drain inserted will have pain and mobility issues. These patients need support to be able to prevent future complications. The most common postoperative complications are bleeding, pneumonia, and wound infection [5]. All postoperative patients are in danger developing a deep vein thrombosis.

To avoid the majority of these complications, it is absolutely mandatory to mobilize these patients as early and as intensely as possible! The following factors should be considered in each patient individually:

8.2.1   Pain Therapy

Sufficient pain management is crucial for sufficient mobilization as well as for pneumonia prevention. After having a chest drain inserted and/or surgery, inadequately controlled pain may restrict breathing and limit mobilization. Coughing and effective physiotherapy are restricted when the patient suffers from pain. Insufficient pain management can lead to under ventilation and subsequent atelectasis as well as the accumulation of exudates leading to pneumonia [5, 10].

An individualized approach to pain management needs to be taken seriously with each patient.

Pain must be assessed prior to analgesic administration. The experience of pain and its intensity is unique to each individual and subjective. If the patient states that he or she is in pain, then the patient has pain and needs to be dealt with appropriately! Pain assessment with the help of rating scales is a well proven method. Self assessment with the help of a numeric rating scale should be the gold standard. If self assessment is not possible (cognitively restricted or in a child), simplified scales with faces can be used. If no individual assessment can be done, tools such as the Behavioral Pain Scale (PBS) on ITS or the Zurich Pain Scale (ZOPA®) can be used to estimate the individual pain intensity. In patients with dementia, special scores are available. The following aspects need to be considered to appropriately and efficiently manage pain:

- Routine assessment of pain intensity in order to evaluate the clinical course
- Assessment at rest and during mobilization
- If rescue medication is needed, the efficacy of this medication has to be checked
- Watch for side effects such as nausea, constipation, and circulatory problems (Ellegast [7]; Gnass [8]; Schmitter et al. [14]).

8.2.2 Mobilization and Physiotherapy

Patient mobilization is limited due to connection to the chest drain system and the need for support. The importance of mobilization needs to be reviewed with the patient as well their his/her need for support. Solutions should be offered to the patient on an individualized basis. The patient must be informed about the fall hazards due to the tubing and system components. If an epidural is being used, potential side effects such as circulatory depression or sensory disturbances must be taken into account. Always remember that chronic diseases and comorbidities may lead to additional mobility limitations.

To prevent complications, the patient should be provided with all options for physiotherapy and mobilization and be motivated by staff to do as much as possible on his/her own. A close collaboration is essential between nurses, physiotherapists, and patients to maximize mobilization and physiotherapy.

8.2.3   Observation

As described above chest drain therapy has potential risks and patients undergoing such therapy need to be observed at regular intervals. In order to recognize complications as early as possible during chest drain therapy (i.e. pneumonia), the following parameters have to be monitored:

- Routine vital sign assessment: Blood pressure, heart rate (arrhythmias occur quite frequently in patients undergoing thoracic surgery), temperature, and respiratory rate.
- Respiratory assessment: Dyspnea, tachypnea, use of accessory respiratory muscles, symptoms of irregular or shallow breathing
- New cough, in particular when related with suspicious sputum, if necessary get a sample.
- Pain assessment with the help of a pain scale, if necessary the administration of medication.

Abnormalities, in particular fever, dyspnea, and the appearance of subcutaneous emphysema need to be reported to the physician in charge and documented appropriately.

8.2.4   *Mental Status*

Patients in the postoperative period, particularly those who are suffering from pain and/or dyspnea, are under mental stress and may be in fear. The fear may be due to a real or an imaginary danger, fear of death, or related to concerns surrounding future therapies and one's physical condition. Therefore it is absolutely mandatory to support patients in these situations and offer them psychological help. One must strive to minimize their pain and to remedy dyspnea. An example of this is if a patient has an episode of dyspnea: the patient should never be left alone and medical/psychological support must be offered.

Very often dyspnea is related to the fear of death. These patients should be supported to feel safe with their medical care and receive updates on their current condition.

The mental status of patients with an underlying oncological disease is even more important and should be in the focus of all members of the therapeutic team. Information should be individually adapted to each patient's situation and delivered so that the patient feels safe. To create an atmosphere of safety, it is helpful to give as much information (i.e. concerning the limitations when having a chest drain) in advance so the patient is able to adapt himself before issues arise. The patients should also be fully briefed about the chest drain and the operation of the drainage system prior to the initiation of any treatment. This can allow for faster acclimation to having a chest drain, the potential for mobilization, and autonomy as well as the feeling of being well informed and prepared. This can lead to a patient that feels safer and believes in the competence of the treatment team.

8.3   Dressing Change

The frequency of routine dressing changes is individualized and related to the standards of the corresponding hospital. There is no standard concerning who does those dressing changes but most are done by the nursing staff. The first routine change should be done no earlier than 48 h postoperatively unless there is an earlier end to chest drain therapy. There is no evidence that routine dressing changes, whatever that interval may be, is superior to a change that is done when needed. The changes should always be carried out under strict aseptic conditions using sterile materials in a correct way and with the No-Touch-technique to prevent wound infection.

Materials for dressing change (Fig. 8.2):

- Sterile compresses, sterile drain compresses (manufactured with a premade slit)
- Plaster or Film to cover the dressings
- Hand and wound sanitizer
- Two pairs of non-sterile gloves
- If necessary a system to resecure the chest tube
- Trash can

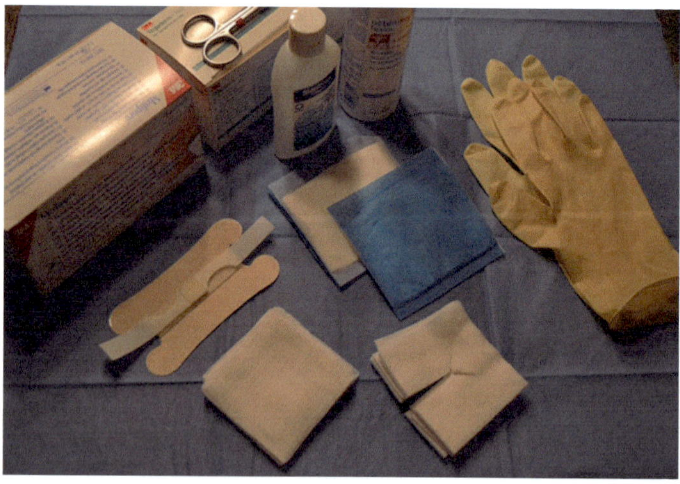

FIGURE 8.2 Materials for dressing change

Procedure:

- Hands should be disinfected before putting on non-sterile gloves. Old dressings are removed and disposed of appropriately. The now dirty gloves are removed and hands disinfected before putting on new gloves.
  Some surgeons place an extra stitch through the skin incision for closing the incision after removal of the chest drain. This extra stitch should not be removed accidently.
- Inspection of the skin incision with regard to erythema, swelling, purulent material, and wideness of the incision: is there a gap between skin and tube?
- Disinfection of the incision: let it interact for 1 min, then dry the wound from the center to the periphery with sterile compresses.
- Put drain dressings (compresses with a slit) around the tube ideally from caudal to cranial and cover these with "normal" compresses. Secure the tube in a way that kinking is prevented.
- Cover the dressing with film or plaster. Remember not to cause too much tension as this can cause tension bullae of the skin. The lack of crinkles is not a sign that the dressing is of correct tightness. Allergies against dressing materials are quite common and must be taken into consideration.
- If necessary, remove the old drainage system to secure the tube then replace it. Watch out for any marks caused by pressure from the tubing pressing on the patient. The tube should be secured in a way that decreases limitations for the patient while also ensuring minimal tension on the skin and potential for clogging.
- If any suspicious findings are seen, these must be documented and reported to the physician in charge (Fig. 8.3).

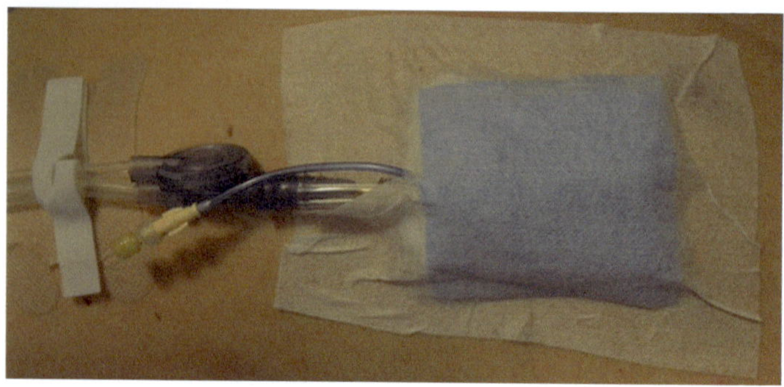

FIGURE 8.3 Dressing with Fixingsystem Secutape® from TechniMed

Literature

1. Bölükbas S, Kudelin N, Dönges T, Schirren J. Therapiemanagement des Chylothorax. Chirurg. 2010;81(3):255–66. doi:10.1007/s00104-009-1858-x.
2. Brunelli A, Salati M, Refai M, Di Nunzio L, Xiumé F, Sabbatini A. Evaluation of a new chest tube removal protocol using digital air leak monitoring after lobectomy: a prospective randomised trial. Eur J Cardiothorac Surg. 2010;37(1):56–60. doi:10.1016/j.ejcts.2009.05.006.
3. Cerfolio RJ, Bryant AS, Skylizard L, Minnich DJ. Optimal technique for the removal of chest tubes after pulmonary resection. J Thorac Cardiovasc Surg. 2013;145(6):1535–9. doi:10.1016/j.jtcvs.2013.02.007.
4. Dango S, Sienel W, Passlick B, Stremmel C. Impact of chest tube clearance on postoperative morbidity after thoracotomy: results of a prospective, randomised trial☆. Eur J Cardiothorac Surg. 2010;37(1):51–5. doi:10.1016/j.ejcts.2009.06.034.
5. Dienemann H. Postoperative Komplikationen in der Thoraxchirurgie. Chirurg. 2009;80(9):807–13. doi:10.1007/s00104-009-1688-x.
6. Eggeling S. Komplikationen in der Therapie des Spontanpneumothorax. Chirurg. 2015;86(5):444–52. doi:10.1007/s00104-014-2866-z.

7. Ellegast J. BASICS Klinische Pharmakologie. 3. Aufl. München: Elsevier, Urban & Fischer (Basics); 2015.
8. Gnass I. Die Schmerzeinschätzung – beobachtet im Intensivbereich. Pflege & Gesellschaft. 2015;20(04):348–61.
9. Halm MA. To strip or not to strip? Physiological effects of chest tube manipulation. Am J Crit Care. 2007;16:609–12.
10. Kiefer T. Thoraxchirurgie. In: Roth M, Kiefer T, Hg. Physiotherapie in der Thoraxchirurgie. Vienna: Springer (SpringerLink: Bücher); 2013, S. 19–40.
11. Linder A. Drainagemanagement nach Lungenresektionen. Zentralbl Chir. 2014;139(S 01):S50–8. doi:10.1055/s-0034-1382923.
12. Refai M, Brunelli A, Salati M, Xiume F, Pompili C, Sabbatini A. The impact of chest tube removal on pain and pulmonary function after pulmonary resection. Eur J Cardiothorac Surg. 2012;41(4):820–3. doi:10.1093/ejcts/ezr126.
13. Saraya T, Light RW, Takizawa H, Goto H. Black pleural effusion. Am J Med. 2013;126(7):641.e1–6. doi:10.1016/j.amjmed.2012.11.017.
14. Schmitter M, List T, Wirz S. Erfassung der Schmerzintensität mit eindimensionalen Skalen. Z Evid Fortbild Qual Gesundhwes. 2013;107(4–5):279–84. doi:10.1016/j.zefq.2013.05.008.
15. Sziklavari Z, Neu R, Hofmann H-S, Ried M. Persistierender Erguss nach thoraxchirurgischen Eingriffen. Chirurg. 2015;86(5):432–6. doi:10.1007/s00104-014-2863-2.

Chapter 9
Management of the Pleural Space: Handling of Chest Tubes and Drainage Systems

Thomas Kiefer

The use of chest tubes and drainage systems has to be an effective treatment and sensible for the patient: this has to be done in reasonable time and without complications to reach the intended goals. Therefore it is crucial to discuss some basic issues that must be remembered as we plan the appropriate settings on the system.

9.1 Pleural Exchange of Fluid and Biomechanics of the Lungs

Depending on body weight and height, anywhere between 2 and 5 ml of pleural fluid are in the pleural space [7]. Under physiological conditions, 15–30 ml/day are produced on each side. Production and reabsorption may be increased up to 500 ml/day with the development of a pleural effusion [10].

T. Kiefer
Chefarzt Klinik für Thoraxchirurgie, Lungenzentrum Bodensee, Klinikum Konstanz, Luisenstr. 7, 78464 Konstanz, Germany
e-mail: Thomas.Kiefer@glkn.de

© Springer International Publishing Switzerland 2017 153
T. Kiefer (ed.), *Chest Drains in Daily Clinical Practice*,
DOI 10.1007/978-3-319-32339-8_9

9.1.1 Fluid Exchange

Pleural fluid is produced and reabsorbed in the parietal pleura. Fluid is filtered by capillaries from the parietal pleura and reabsorbed by lymphatic vessels.

The influence of gravitation pressure applied to the fluid (=pressure in the pleural space), presuming an upright or sitting position, is increased with height (i.e. getting "more subatmospheric"). Pressure is ± 0 cm H_2O at the level of the diaphragm and about 10 cm H_2O at the level of the heart.

9.1.2 Biomechanics of the Lungs

The pressure in the pleural space is larger than the elastic recoil of the lung. This pressure difference along with the adhesive forces caused by the pleural fluid, cause the lung to remain expanded in the chest cavity.

The elastic recoil forces can be approximately measured via the transesophageal pressure. At the level of the heart this is about 4 cm H_2O. It is less (=less negative) in an emphysematous lung and higher (=more negative) with a fibrotic lung [12].

During inspiration, the diameter of the chest is increased causing an increase in intrathoracic volume. Due to adhesive forces, the lung has to follow the chest wall therefore causing an increase in the "negative pressure" in the pleural space.

During expiration this "negative pressure" decreases. As gravity is also involved, this subatmospheric pressure is highest at the end of inspiration at the tip of the lung (=pleural cupola) and lowest at the end of expiration down at the diaphragm in an upright or seated position. Approximate measures of the pleural pressure show pressures ranging from zero to minus 15 cm of water. This physiological data should always be kept in mind as we think about pressure settings of the corresponding drainage system.

9.1.3   Changes in Pleural Respiratory Function After Lung Resection

When reviewing the changes in respiratory function after lung resection, one must differentiate between the early and late postoperative changes. The amount of lung resected as well as the surgical approach to the chest cavity play an important roll. All kinds of thoracotomies are correlated in the early postoperative period with a limitation of inspiration and expiration that is mainly pain related but also functional in nature. Later in the postoperative course, a mainly restrictive disturbance of ventilation is seen caused by scarring in the areas of incisions and sometimes the parietal pleura. The latter is more impressive the larger the size of the thoracotomy.

Pleural manipulation will always result in fluid production. This may lead to the development of a pleural effusion if the chest drain treatment was inefficient or if the tube was removed too early [3].

9.1.4   Drainage of the Pleural Cavity After Lung Operations

Immediately after closure of the chest, the main goal of the chest tube is to evacuate air from the thoracic cavity.

Compliance ($\Delta V/\Delta P$) of the lung decreases proportionally with resected lung volume [11].

According to theoretical pathophysiological considerations, there is a danger of acute hyperinflation if the lung is brought up too fast postoperatively. Parenchymal injuries with laceration of the alveoli could occur resulting in a lung edema or ARDS [16].

In clinical reality, this rarely occurs or its consequences do not become obvious. As the diaphragm elevates on the side of the resection, this volume reduction prevents hyperinflation. A relative diaphragmatic elevation will be observed in most cases after a significant loss of lung tissue.

Reexpansion pulmonary edema is fortunately a rare entity that is seen after drainage of a complete pneumothorax or a large pleural effusion. This is probably related to injury of the aleolar walls and the release of toxic mediators after reperfusion of previously nonventilated and nonperfused areas [15].

9.2   Management of the Pleural Space

The goal of the chest drain treatment is the restoration of physiological conditions in the pleural space.

At first glance this phrase may not impress much, but it is important and should be the basis of all considerations when dealing with a chest drain.

"Restoration of physiological conditions in the pleural space" means that we follow these conditions as we, for example, set a pressure in the drainage system (i.e. generating a subatmospheric pressure in the pleural space). This also means that we have to clarify when we have reached the criteria for chest tube removal, particularly when monitoring chest tube output.

9.2.1   Number of Drains

There is consensus that one chest tube is sufficient for the treatment of a pneumothorax as well as of a simple, free-floating effusion.

It was common practice worldwide in the few past decades to use two (or even three) chest tubes after an anatomical resection. In the recent years, a trend has emerged to use just one drain after these procedures. Numerous studies [1, 2, 5, 13, 16] have shown that regardless of which lobe has been resected, using only one chest tube results in equivalent or better pain control, shorter lengths of stay, and lower costs as compared to two or more.

In most postoperative situations one chest tube is sufficient. This is true for all anatomical and extraanatomical lung resections.

9.2.2   Start of Chest Drain Treatment

9.2.2.1   Postoperatively

After closing the chest and placing dressings, the chest tube is connected to the drainage system. When using an electronic system, the default standard settings automatically start when it is turned on.

9.2.2.2   Post Intervention

It has been pointed out several times that the risk for developing reexpansion pulmonary edema is in particularly high when a pneumothorax or large effusion preexists for a longer time period (>4 days). Reexpansion of the lung has to be performed according to the clinical situation even if these entities have existed for just a short while. The old rule to not drain more than one liter per day is no longer valid. The focus should be focused on the patient's cardiopulmonary status. Quite often during reinflation of the lung, a nagging cough that is refractory to treatment is observed. This is another reason to be careful when draining effusions and wait to apply subatmospheric pressure until the lung has appropriately reinflated passively. Individual experience and clinical judgment are needed in these situations as well as the empathy to share knowledge and experience with one's young colleagues!

9.2.3   Drainage System Settings

When using water seal, in this instance meaning a one chamber system, it is mandatory to keep the canister positioned below the chest. Furthermore the stab of the water seal has to be pulled out of the fluid as the fluid level rises. If this is not done the patient is no longer able to actively evacuate air from a parenchymal leak from the chest cavity when a distinct fluid level is reached. This will result in a pneumothorax and/or subcutaneous emphysema.

When active (=external) suction is used, most often a subatmospheric pressure of −15 to −20 cm of water is set. Once more it has to be emphasized that in conventional, commercially manufactured multichamber systems (i.e. "historic" bottle systems or newer one, two, or three chamber systems) only the pressure in the system is known and can be regulated. The intrapleural pressure of which we are ultimately interested is not directly monitored. It is only possible to measure, or nearly to measure, with electronic regulated systems, where the pressure is measured next to the patient comparing that value with set value (see Chap. 5).

Different clinical situations and diseases may need variations in settings from what is the standard. After lung resection or even lung volume reduction in bullous emphysema there is a tendency towards the application of minimal subatmospheric pressure or even a Heimlich valve. In these particular situations a provider with clinical experience, intuition, and the empathy cannot fall into activism

There are multiple clinical situations where an increase in the subatmospheric pressure may be indicated to mechanically drive the expansion of the lung. Such a situation could be after a decortication for empyema or after bilobectomy. There is no data that such a procedure has a repeatable, positive effect.

Linder [8] described the concept of parenchymal fistulas that may open and close. This consideration assumes that some parenchymal leaks will close with increased subatmospheric pressure while others will get bigger. A therapeutic algorithm has not become reality to date in reference to this.

Refai et al. [14] described applying different subatmospheric pressure settings according to the anatomic lung resection (i.e. right upper lobectomy vs. left lower lobectomy) but was not embraced in the broader surgeon community.

9.2.4 Duration of Treatment

The moment of chest drainage cessation is the same as the moment the chest tube is pulled. In the postoperative setting following standard lung resection this is defined as the time where the patient meets the medical center's criteria for chest tube removal. In all other indications, the chest tube is removed after reaching the predefined therapeutic goals (see Chap. 3).

9.2.4.1   Treatment After Standard Lung Resections

Following anatomical and extra anatomic resections, the chest tube will be removed when the hospital's criteria concerning air leak and fluid production are fulfilled (see also Chap. 12). The timing since surgery should not be an issue when the indication for chest tube removal is met.

9.2.4.2   Pneumothorax

When a pneumothorax is treated with surgery, usually a thorascopic approach is used and the same rules apply as in standard resections (see above).

There is no valid, evidence based data concerning the duration of conservative treatment of a spontaneous pneumothorax [2, 9]. After chest tube insertion and quick resolution of air leaks, chest tube therapy will typically last 48–72 h in most centers.

When a pneumothorax is initially treated conservatively, an electronic system may be helpful as objective data concerning flow representing the quantity of a parenchymal leak is provided.

After the insertion of a chest tube for a spontaneous pneumothorax, a subatmospheric pressure in the pleural space generated by gentle suction usually shows a flow that will rapidly decrease and reach zero (=no parenchymal leak.)

When a parenchymal leak with a flow of >100 ml/min for a couple hours is seen after initiating treatment, it is the author's opinion that the patient should be informed that an expeditious operation would be beneficial. In such a situation, it is common to find at least one ruptured bulla intraoperatively. The healing of such a bullae takes, if anything, a long time as compared to a surgical approach where a postoperative stay is typically one to three days. Thanks to this strategy, chest tube drainage time and length of hospital stay can be reduced significantly.

9.2.4.3   Pleurodesis

After pleurodesis, which is most often completed with thorascopic talc application, (see also Chap. 3) the only criterion for treatment completion is based on fluid production. The lung should be more or less fully expanded as otherwise a pleurodesis wouldn't have been indicated. There is no evidence based data to guide when to remove the chest tube in these patients. According to the author's own experience, the drain can be removed safely when fluid production is below 100 ml/day.

9.2.4.4   Pleural Empyema

Whether treatment of a pleural empyema is conservative or surgical, the goals therapy are the same: complete and permanent control of the underlying inflammatory/infectious disease, more or less complete inflation of the lung, and the removal of all fluid compartments. An air leak in the setting of an empyema, especially after a surgical pleurectomy/decortication should be taken into account when deciding on chest tube removal. Relevant parameters that would allow for the safe removal of the chest tube(s) are:

- Repeated proof of freedom of microbes in the drained fluid (i.e. when there had been positive findings initially)
- More or less complete inflation of the lung
- Removal of all fluid compartments
- Inflammatory parameters in the blood analysis are normal (as long as there is no other explanation)

The guidelines for the treatment of pleural empyemas [4] are very vague in regard to the duration of treatment. This is due to the heterogeneity of this disease making it nearly impossible to give universal and evidence based advice.

9.3   Interpretation of Air Leaks

The difficulty to change from a conventional bottle or canister system with a water seal to an electronic system that objectively measures air leaks and acquires data is mostly cultural (i.e. cultural shock)

When the use of electronic systems started there was tentativeness likely due initial difficulty in interpreting data and knowing, for example, what a flow of 100 ml/min means. Today after more than seven years of use and thousands of therapeutic procedures where these systems have been utilized we are able to classify the data presented on the screen and draw the right conclusions (Table 9.1). It has to be emphasised that data interpretation is purely empiric as valid, evidence based data is not available to date!

The interpretation of data and the subsequent conclusions made must always be done in the context of the underlying disease, the condition of the lung ("normal"; emphysematous, fibrotic), surgery or intervention performed, and the duration of therapy so far. Remember that healing is a dynamic process!

Another advantage of electronic system, besides the generation of objective data, is the capability to recall previous data on the screens (Fig. 9.1) allowing for evaluation over time at a glance. This is compared to traditional systems where decisions are made "statically" during morning or evening rounds.

The interpretation of data acquired from an electronic drainage system should be placed in the context of the underlying disease, condition of the lung, procedure, and duration of therapy.

TABLE 9.1 Interpretation of postoperative objectively acquired flow data

Description of leak	Objectively measured data	Therapeutic consequence
Not tolerable	≥3000 ml/min	Immediately postop "Normal"lung: sudden reexploration Emphysematous lung: wait for 1–2 days then revision if no trend towards healing
Very large	1500–3000 ml/min	Wait if trend towards healing is observed, otherwise quick revision
Large	500–1500 ml/min	>500 ml/min constantly over more than 7 days: revision
Small leak	50–500 ml/min	Correction of the tube If necessary: Heimlich-Valve
No leak	≤40 ml/min constantly over 6 h	Pull the drain

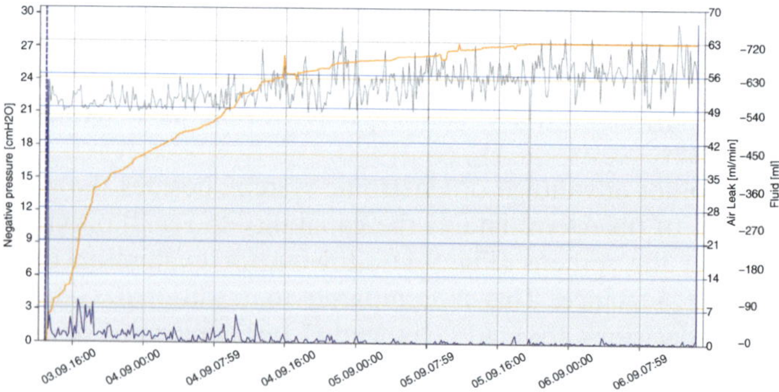

FIGURE 9.1 Display flow (*grey*: subatmospheric pressure, *blue*: flow, *yellow*: fluid production)

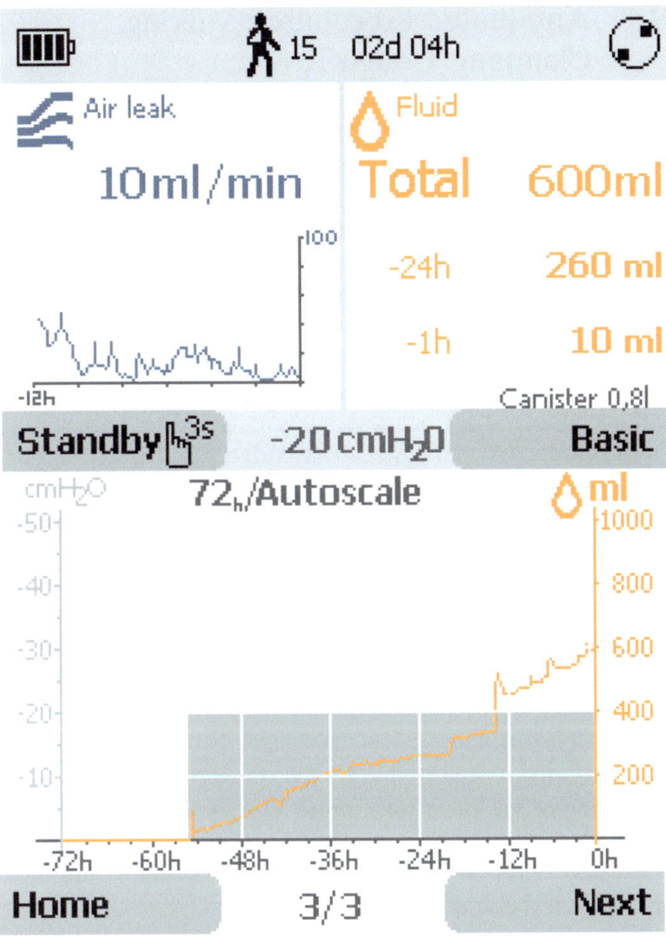

FIGURE 9.2 Display fluid

The author is well aware that this proposal of how to interpret objective data consists of haziness and conclusions drawn that are due to clinical experience and not based on evidence. At the end of the day every physician has to make decisions based on his/her own experience (see below).

9.4   Antiquated Procedures: Milking, Clamping, Cough Test

9.4.1   Milking or Stripping

This is a widely done procedure to prevent clogging of the intrathoracic tube which is not visible and thus cannot be observed. In times of modern electronic drainage systems that are able to show patency of the tube on the screen (one manufacturer), prophylactic milking and stripping is obsolete. Additionally there is no proven benefit with regard to patency rates. Several authors have shown this inefficacy [6, 17]. The latter conducted a Cochrane analysis including only studies from centers that perform cardiac surgery. In cardiac surgery the problem of tube clogging is much more evident as compared to thoracic surgery. In addition, unpredictable high pressure of up to -400 cm of water can be provoked during the milking process which could lead to parenchymal injury.

Prophylactic milking or stripping of chest drains is ineffective and can be dangerous, and thus it is obsolete.

9.4.2   Clamping

Clamping of the chest tube, up to 24 h, is also a widely used procedure, This is performed to increase the success of the chest drain therapy ending and therefore bringing the decision to pull the drain to a solid base.

This is dangerous! Clamping a chest drain is simulating a clinical setting with no tube. Doing so there is no chance to control and observe what is going on inside the chest cavity and the pleural space respectively. In particular, such a procedure can induce significant clinical problems especially if the patients are not monitored very closely. In addition clamping leads to a delay in removal.

With the help of electronic systems all relevant data needed for the decision process for pulling the tube is provided.

Clamping of the chest drain prior to removal is redundant and may be dangerous. In addition it leads to unneeded delay of the removal of the chest tube as well as to an increase in length of stay.

9.4.3   Cough Test

A cough test is performed to assess adequate that an adequate seal has formed in the lung parenchyma. The patient is asked, when using a classic drainage system with water seal, to cough firmly. If bubbles are observed in the collection chamber of the system this is taken as "confirmation" of an ongoing leak.

Again this procedure is as widely used and senseless! It is almost always possible to mobilize some bubble when coughing. These bubble are "responsible" for the chest tube not being pulled. Additionally in patients with severe emphysema this procedure may be problematic.

This is another situation where a modern electronic system would provide very sensitive data and be able to detect the smallest leaks with objective data. It allows all necessary information at the moment and over the time to pull the chest tube on time, safely, and without unnecessary delay. Remember that healing is a dynamic process!

9.5   Drainage After Pneumonectomy

The discussion of whether to drain the chest cavity after pneumonectomy or not comes coming up from time to time. There are no guidelines nor clinical studies concerning this issue that would allow to finish this discussion based on evidence based scientific data.

Some thoracic surgeons do not drain the chest cavity after pneumonectomy. Others insert one chest tube that is clamped, removing this clamp from time to time to monitor fluid production (and blood loss) for the first 12–24 h. In my own practice, the clamp is opened every hour and the drain is removed in an uneventful course after 12–14 h.

It can be dangerous to let the drain open towards the atmosphere or apply a subatmospheric pressure by a suction source to the chest cavity after pneumonectomy. These maneuvers can lead to life threatening mediastinal shift towards the side of operation. Symptoms are the same as in a tension pneumothorax: the large veins of the upper part of the body can kink leading to a low cardiac input syndrome followed by circulatory depression, superior vena cava syndrome, and anxiety for the patient.

Even a very gentle subatmospheric pressure can induce this described cascade. Mediastinal shift can also occur in the presence or absence of a (clamped) drain in particular in the first hours after surgery. In such a situation it can be helpful to open the drain towards atmosphere, let the patient take some deep breaths to relocate the mediastinum.

After pneumonectomy it may be dangerous to let the chest tube open towards the atmosphere or to apply subatmospheric pressure. This might provoke symptoms and consequences comparable with those seen in a tension pneumothorax.

9.6   Ventilated Patient

A patient on a ventilator who has a chest drain, regardless of the indication, does not need an active suction source. The ventilator presses air via the trachea and bronchi through the parenchyma into the pleural space (in the presence of a parenchymal leak) and from there through the chest drain(s) outside of the chest cavity.

As a patient on the ventilator develops subcutaneous emphysema (Fig. 9.3) the solution in most cases is not the generation of a subatmospheric pressure but correct positioning of the drain(s). In general it has to be warned against activism and the placement of numerous chest tubes. One or two

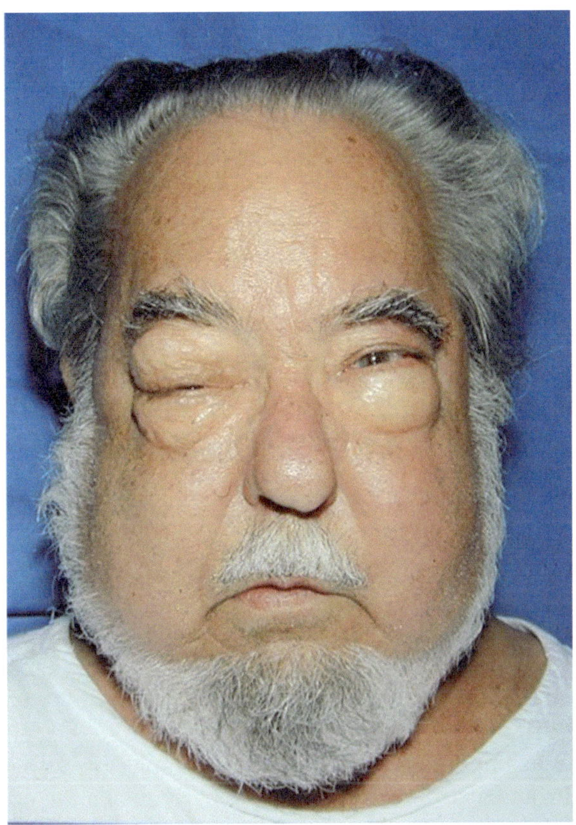

FIGURE 9.3 Subcutaneous emphysema

chest tubes in adequate position combined with patience in both the patient and physician will solve the problem in almost all cases.

9.7   Myths

When discussing chest drains, chest drain systems, and their management, there are inevitably some myths that will come up that need to be dismissed:

9.7.1   Myth No. 1: Water Seal Is "No Suction"

The Heber-Principle is based exactly on the opposite of this statement! This principle uses the height difference of two compartments, here the pleural space and the collection chamber of the system, and a tube filled with fluid. The sub-atmospheric pressure that results in the pleural space correlates in daily clinical life to the height difference from bed to floor which is normally around 60 cm. Any physician hardly would apply such a "negative" pressure on purpose!

9.7.2   Myth No. 2: Parenchymal Leaks Heal Faster Without Suction

Almost all of the protagonists that keep this myth alive use a water seal modality in the sense of the Heber principle. The myth that a relatively high subatmospheric pressure in the pleural space causing longer air leaks can be rebutted by a simple and impressive example given by Alex Brunelli:

When one drinks a soft drink though a straw, a certain amount of fluid is obtained. If you suck harder, you'll get more of the drink but did the diameter of the straw get bigger?

This example can be illustrated by a graph (Fig. 9.4) generated by an electronic drainage system: Reducing the applied pressure reduces the flow (=parenchymal leak). This is no hint for healing!

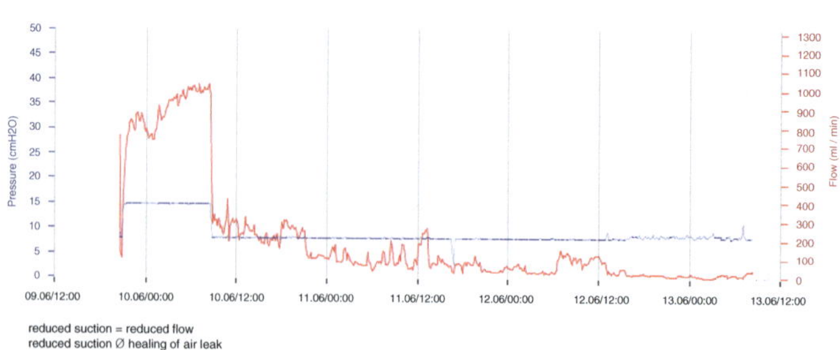

FIGURE 9.4 Correlation suction and flow. Reduced suction = reduced flow, reduced suction Ø healing of air leak (Data provided courtesy of Alex Brunelli, Leeds)

Literature

1. Alex J, Ansari J, Bahalkar P, et al. Comparisom of immediate postoperative outcome of using conventional two drains versus a single drain after lobectomy. Ann Thorac Surg. 2003;76(4): 1056–9.
2. Baumann M, Strange C, Heffner J, et al. Management of spontaneous pneumothorax. An American College of Chest Physicians Delphi consensus statement. Chest. 2001;119:590–602.
3. Brunelli A, Beretta E, Cassivi SD, Cerfolio RJ, Detterbeck F, Kiefer T, et al. Consensus definitions to promote an evidence-based approach to management of the pleural space. A collaborative proposal by ESTS, AATS, STS and GTSC. Eur J Cardiothorac Surg. 2011;40(2011):291–7.
4. Davies HE, Davies RJO, Davies CWH. Management of pleural infection in adults: British Thoracic Society pleural disease guideline 2010. Thorax. 2010;65(Suppl 2):ii41–53. doi:10.1136/thx2010.137026.
5. Gómez-Caro A, Roca MJ, Torres J, et al. Successful use of a single chest drain postlobectomy instead of two classical drains: a randomized study. Eur J Cardiothorac Surg. 2006;29(4):562–6.
6. Halm MA. To strip or not to strip? Physiological effects of chest tube manipulation. Am J Crit Care. 2007;16(6):609–12.
7. Haverkamp W, Herth F, Messmann H. Internistische Intensivmedizin. Stuttgart: Thieme; 2008.
8. Linder A. Thoraxdrainagen und Drainagesystem – Moderne Konzepte. UNI-MED Verlag; 2014.
9. MacDuff A, Arnold A, Harvey J, on behalf of the BTS Pleural Disease Guideline Group. Management of spontaneous pneumothorax: British Thoracic Society pleural disease guideline. Chest. 2010;119:590–602.
10. Matthys H, Seeger W. Klinische Pneumologie. 4. Aufl. Berlin: Springer; 2008.
11. Miserocchi G, Negrini D. Pleural space: pressure and fluid dynamics. In: Crystal RG, editor. The lunge: Scientific Foundations. New York: Raven Press; 1977. p. 1217–25.
12. Miserocchi G, Beretta E, Rivolta I. Respiratory mechanics and fluid dynamics after lung resection surgery. Thorac Surg Clin. 2010;20(3):345–57.
13. Okur E, Baysungur V, Tezel C, et al. Comparison of the single or double chest tube applications after pulmonary lobectomies. Eur J Cardiothorac Surg. 2009;35(1):32–5.
14. Refai M, Brunelli A, Varela G, Novoa N, Pompili C, Jimenez MF, Aranda JL, Sabbatini A. The values of intrapleural pressure

before removal of chest tube in non-complicated pulmonary lobectomies. Eur J Cardiothorac Surg. 2012:1–3.

15. Rozeman J, Yellin A, Simansky DA, Shiner RJ. Re-expansion pulmonary oedema following spontaneous pneumothorax. Respir Med. 1996;90:235–8.

16. Tattersall DJ, Traill ZC, Gleeson FV. Chest drains: does size matters? Clin Radiol. 2000;55(6):415–21.

17. Wallen MA, Morrison AL, Gillies D, O'Riordan E, Bridge C, Stoddart F. Mediastinal chest drain clearance for cardiac surgery (Review). The Cochrane Library. 2010;(7).

Chapter 10
Pain Management in Patients with a Chest Drain

Dana Mergner

10.1 Systemic Pain Management

There are different approaches to drug administration in patients with a chest drain: oral, parenteral (subcutaneous or iv), or rectal. Oral medications ("by mouth") are preferred however the route of application is mainly determined by the severity of pain and the possibility of enteral absorption. In the (early) post operative period, patients may suffer from nausea, vomiting, and from gastroenteral atony. In these cases, IV application is preferred (IV, PCA, short infusion).

When very severe pain is encountered, the drug of choice is an opioid. There are several very potent opioids (morphine, hydromorphone, fentanyl, sufentanil, piritramide, pethidine) and low potency opioids (tramadol, tilidine/naloxone) to choose from which should be used according to the experience of the physician and the individual circumstances of the patient.

D. Mergner
Sektionsleiterin Schmerztherapie, Klinikum Konstanz,
Luisenstr. 7, 78464 Constance, Germany
e-mail: Dana.Mergner@glkn.de

© Springer International Publishing Switzerland 2017
T. Kiefer (ed.), *Chest Drains in Daily Clinical Practice*,
DOI 10.1007/978-3-319-32339-8_10

In addition nonopioid medications such as NSAIDS (diclofenac, ibuprofen), COX2 inhibitors, paracetamol or metamizol can be added to the pain management according to the WHO analgesic ladder [5].

10.1.1   IV PCA

Administering pain medication intravenously allows for analgesia to be achieved much faster. Patients with a chest drain have often undergone major surgery which causes even more pain compared with "just the chest drain". In cases of severe pain, early postoperative patient controlled analgesia is a better way of achieving efficient analgesia as compared to other conventional modalities (subcutaneous, or short infusion). In patients that have never before received opioids, drug administration should to be done by intermittent bolus as continuous application could lead to respiratory depression.

10.1.2   Oral Opioids

Opioids are synthetically produced drugs with a morphine like effect and cause effective analgesia by linking to central and peripheral opioid receptors. Typical side effects of opioids include: respiratory depression, tiredness, dizziness, sedation, nausea, vomiting, constipation, and development of tolerance.

Like in post-operative pain-management, opioids are the drug of first choice in severe pain management caused by a chest drain alone. Oral administration of a retarded opioid as a baseline analgesia combined with a non-retarded opioid if necessary represents an efficient concept. To use this concept in an optimal way an algorithm should be developed to allow drug administration on demand without reconfirmation by the physician in charge [2].

10.1.3   Non-opioid Analgesics

In addition to opioids, nonopioid analgesics should be given as baseline medication to achieve balanced analgesia. Using a combination of medications with different mechanisms of action causes improved pain reduction, a decrease in opioid doses, and a decrease in side effects of each drug.

10.1.4   Nonopioid Analgesics

Metamizol

Positive: No hepatic, renal, or gastrointestinal side effects.
Negative: Intolerances and circulatory reactions may occur as unintended side effects. A rate of agranulocytosis of 1:30,000 – 1:500,000 is reported in the literature.

Paracetamol

There is an insignificant reduction in opioid dosages and no reduction in opioid related side effects. The most dangerous side effect is hepatic toxicity which can occur when administered above daily dose limits.

NSAIDs and Caribe

Positive: NSAIDs have analgesic, antiphlogistic and antipyretic effects.
Negative: Main side effects are gastrointestinal ones, acute kidney failure, and cardiovascular complications.

Co-analgesics

Pain caused by a chest drain is typically neuropathic in nature with a sharp and burning quality due to the irritation of an intercostal nerve. Therefore pain medication should always include drugs that have an effect on neuropathic pain.

The best ratio of side effects versus activity profile for neuropathic pain are anticonvulsive drugs (i.e. pregabalin and gabapentin). Both drugs have an effect on the $\alpha2$-δ-unit of tension dependent Ca channels and reduce the inflow of calcium into the nerve cell. Pregabalin also has an anxiolytic effect and supports sleep (Baron).

10.2   Regional Anesthesia

10.2.1   Epidural Anesthesia

Thoracic epidural anesthesia is the most effective method to treat discomfort in patients with chest tubes. Epidural anesthesia is a regional treatment that administers local anesthetic close to the spinal cord in the epidural space, frequently in combination with an opioid and/or a $\alpha2$-adrenergic receptor agonist. Epidural catheters are placed between T4 and T10 in order to achieve appropriate pain control regarding the chest drain. This medication can be administered as a one time single injection into the epidural space or as a continuous infusion using a catheter.

Contraindications for epidural anesthesia include a patient refusing the method, coagulopathy, infection in the area of injection, and allergies to local anesthetics.

Several side effects and complications may occur during epidural anesthesia:

- A block of the sympathetic nerve or parts of the nerve may lead to a significant decrease in blood pressure which requires treatment.
- During puncture, an injury to the dura mater by the needle can occur which can cause a "spinal" headache.
- If local anesthetic is incorrectly infused in a spinal location, hypotension, respiratory depression, and significant bradycardia may occur.

- The spinal cord may be injured if the site of puncture is too high, which can lead to neuropathic pain and signs of paralysis.
- Injury to blood vessels in the epidural space can result in a hematoma causing pressure on the spinal cord with subsequent neurological symptoms (even paraplegia).
- A severe complication is an epidural abscess as a result of a non sterile procedure or the hematogenous spread from a neighboring infected area. This can also lead to neurological deficits to include paraplegia.
- Systemic side effects of the local anesthetic can include neuro and/or cardiotoxic symptoms.

Administration of the drugs (opioid and/or local anesthetics) can also be done by a patient controlled system (patient controlled epidural application) which results in a better efficiency of pain control and a better tractability by the patient.

10.2.2   Paravertebral Block

A paravertebral block is a procedure comparable to epidural analgesia in efficiency but has less side effects. Therefore a paravertebral block may be a very good procedure to treat pain in patients with chest drains.

The paravertebral space is a triangular space which is bordered by the vertebral body (lateral), pleura (anterior), lig. costotransversum (posterior), and the vertebral body (medial). The spinal nerve with ramus ventralis and dorsalis as well as pre and postganglionic fibers of the sympathetic trunk are located there. Applying local anesthesic here causes an unilateral sympathetic, motor, and sensory block.

Side effects and complications of paravertebral blocks include:

- Pneumothorax can occur due to unintended injury to the pleura. This can be less dramatic if there is already a chest tube in place.

- Horner syndrome can occur due to block of the stellate ganglion located at the level of the first thoracic vertebra (rare).
- Unintended puncture of the dura leads to spinal anaesthesia
- Unintended injection of local anesthetic may lead to cardiac (arrhythmia) and/or neurological (cerebral seizure) complications.
- Allergic reactions to local anesthetics can occur.
- As in all other regional anesthetic procedures, there may be no effect on pain control.

Paravertebral blocks are infrequently used as it is not an easy procedure.

How to Do a Paravertebral Block

- Lateral decubitus position with the side of interest upwards.
- Puncture 3 cm cranial to the target spinal process in the median line with a local anesthetic using a 10 cm long needle for stimulation.
- Position the needle at a 90° angle to the skin. After approximately 4 cm, bone contact with the transverse process is had.
- Now the needle will be withdrawn just underneath the skin and a 10° angle is made cranially.
- The needle is cautiously pushed forward with the help of the resistance loss technique (with air) max. 1.5 cm more than the bone contact marker.
- After the loss of resistance and negative aspiration, a local anaesthetic is injected (i.e. 20 ml ropivacaine 0.75 %).

10.2.3 Intercostal Nerve Block

An intercostal nerve block is another option of peripheral regional anesthesia. Intercostal nerves derive from the rami ventrales from the corresponding spinal nerves on each side of all thoracic vertebrae. They run along the lower edge of the ribs with the corresponding artery and vein, between the external and internal intercostal muscles and part of the abdominal muscles. The nerves innervate the intercostal muscles and are responsible for one segment of sensory innervation.

The nerve block at the level of the chest drain skin incision allows precise analgesia of the corresponding intercostal nerve. Chest drains are usually inserted between the third and sixth intercostal spaces in the anterior or midaxillary line. The block will be performed at the corresponding level.

This method can be utilized to treat the potential severe pain that occurs after insertion a chest drain or intra or pre-operatively for thoracotomy or thoracoscopy.

Contraindications include: patient refusal, coagulopathy, infection in the area of puncture, or allergies to local anes-thetics. Remember that the accumulation of local anesthetics may lead to arrhythmias, acute myocardial infarction, and to epilepsy.

Due to the close approximation of the intercostal artery and vein, there is the possibility for systemic uptake of the local anesthetic followed by cardiac complications (arrhyth-mia) or cerebral dysfunction (cerebral seizure). Another complication with these transcutaneous blocks is a pneumo-thorax. As the procedure is carried out to solve pain caused by a chest drain, this complication can be neglected as a drain is already in place.

How to Do an Intercostal Nerve Block

- This can be performed in a sitting position (Angelus Costae) or in a lateral decubitus position the arm above the head (posterior axillary line).
- The lower edge of the rib is identified. After proper skin disinfection the skin is anesthezised with local anesthetic.
- The skin above the corresponding rib is pulled gently cra-nially and a needle (25G) is directed towards the lower edge of the rib until the rib is reached.

- After contact with the rib, the tension on the skin is released and the needle is gently pushed forward under the rib for 2–3 mm. In order not to cause a pneumothorax, the needle should not be driven forward any further.
- 4–6 ml of a local anesthetic is injected (i.e. ropivacaine 0.75 %).
- As the region innervated by a single intercostal nerve overlaps the segment above and below, the skin incision should also be anesthesized by this block.

10.3   Patients Treated with a Chest Drain Without Surgery

Patients with a chest drain that did not undergo surgery (i.e. first event of a spontaneous pneumothorax) tend to suffer less pain. A regional anesthesic is indicated as there are less systemic side effects. If contraindications exist or the patient denies this time of anesthesia, pain control should be performed according the WHO staging scheme. Whenever possible physiotherapy should be added.

10.4   Patients with a History of Opioid Dependence

In patients that are opioid dependent or formerly dependent, regional anesthesia is preferred as long as there are no specific contraindications and the patient is amenable. In addition nonopioids and coanalgesics should be administered to optimize pain management.

Opioids can also be administered in patients with a history of opioid dependence according to their pain intensity. According to the WHO staging scheme, therapy should be started with a low potency opioid (tilidine, naloxone). If needed these drugs might be replaced by a high potent opioid. If necessary a long lasting medication can be administered.

Insufficient pain control in a patient suffering from addiction must be avoided.

10.5   Application of Lidocaine Gel

To reduce pain caused by a chest drain, lidocaine gel (2 %) is applied as to cover the skin incision and the area where the tubing is in contact with the skin [1].

Literature

1. Kang H, Chung YS, Choe JW, Woo YC, Kim SW, Park SJ, et al. Application of lidocaine jelly on chest tubes to reduce pain caused by drainage catheter after coronary artery bypass surgery. J Korean Med Sci. 2014;29(10):1398–403.
2. Pogatzki-Zahn E. Update postoperative Schmerztherapie, Refresher Course Nr. 39. April 2013.
3. S1-Leitlinie. Pharmakologisch nicht interventionelle Therapie chronisch neuropathischer Schmerzen, AWMF-Registernummer: 030/114. Baron, R. Leitlinien für Diagnostik und Therapie in der Neurologie.
4. S3-Leitlinie. Behandlung akuter perioperativer und posttraumatischer Schmerzen, AWMF-Register Nr. 041/001. Stand: 21.05.2007, inkl. Änderungen vom 20.04.2009.
5. Vargas-Schaffer G. Is the WHO analgesic ladder still valid? Twenty-four years of experience. Can Fam Physician. 2010;56(6): 514–7.

Chapter 11
Physiotherapy in Patients with Chest Drains

Kathrin Süss

The question of whether all patients with a chest drain need physiotherapy (physical therapy) is a controversial issue. The author feels that the checklist below helps to determine if physiotherapy is indicated. If any one of the questions is answered "yes" the patient should have physiotherapy. The checklist is intentionally kept simple without focusing on the underlying disease that led to chest drain therapy. The list that follows reviews the general consequences of a chest drain.

1. Insufficient mobility: yes/no
2. Pain change with change in posture: yes/no
3. Poor respiratory effort: yes/no
4. Dyspnea: yes/no
5. Delirium/Dementia: yes/no

K. Süss
Asklepios Fachkliniken München-Gauting,
Robert-Koch-Alle 2, 82131 Gauting, Germany
e-mail: k.suess@asklepios.com

© Springer International Publishing Switzerland 2017
T. Kiefer (ed.), *Chest Drains in Daily Clinical Practice*,
DOI 10.1007/978-3-319-32339-8_11

11.1   Insufficient Mobility

A patient's mobility can be improved with ambulation training. Answering the following questions makes planning such training more effective:

1. Is ambulation training only possible with the support of a physiotherapist?
2. Is ambulation training indicated due to respiratory aspects?
3. Is a walker/walking frame needed?

One goal of ambulation training is the optimization of the patient's self evaluation of walking speed and the timing of breaks. Close collaboration with social workers and case managers is important in order to clarify the patient's home situation (i.e. lives alone, stairs to climb, dependent on oxygen, need for assistance with activities of daily living – ADL training) (Fig. 11.1).

11.2   Pain

The physiotherapist can aid in reduction and/or elimination of pain by contributing the following strategies:

1. Classic massage to reduce muscle tone; "breath stimulation" ointments
2. TENS (Transcutaneous Electric Nerve Stimulation)/Taping
3. Relaxing procedures:

    - Qi Gong/Meditation
    - Feldenkrais
    - Osteopathy, etc.

11.3   Secretion Elimination

- Humid NaCl inhalation (may need to be highly concentrated), or with salbutamol (improves the mucociliary clearance)

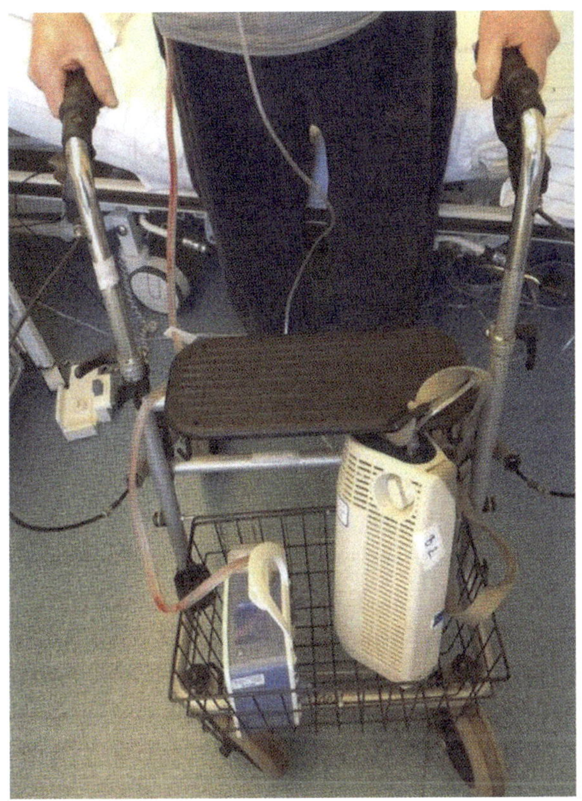

FIGURE 11.1 ADL-training with the help of a walking frame

– Respiratory therapy using Modified Autogenic Drainage (MAD). This method was developed in Belgium for secretion management in Cystic fibrosis patients. The method had been modified in Germany by Rita Kieselmann in order to apply this method to all diseases with secretion retention. The patient is supposed to continue with therapy after instruction by a physiotherapist. If necessary the treatment is combined with inhalation by a PEP (Positive-expiratory Pressure) system. The main principle is based on fluctuation in caliber of the bronchi during inhalation and expiration. See also PEP-systems.

FIGURE 11.2
PEP-system with
oscillation (VRP
1) (Roth and
Kiefer 2013)
(Medtronic
Germany)

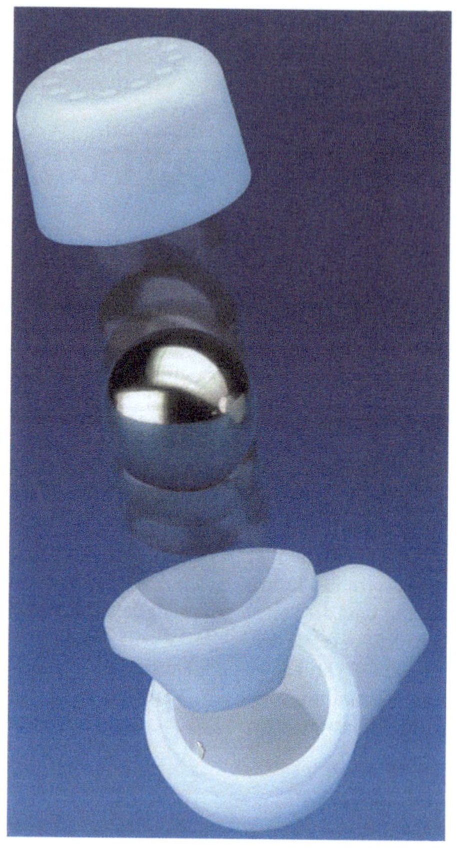

- Positive-expiratory Pressure (PEP) systems (with and without oscillation) can optimizie the utilization of low end pressure in the bronchial system. Simplified: The more peripheral the secretions are located, the deeper the patient has to inhale to bring air behind the secretion. The pause at the end of inspiration is supposed to open blood vessel collaterals minimizing mismatches in perfusion. Expiration is used for further secretion transportation towards the centrally located airways. As secretions are moved more centrally, the shorter the inspiration needed and the longer the expiration required to further transport the secretions towards the throat (Fig. 11.2).

Remark

In the physiotherapist's community, there is ongoing discussions on whether technique highlighting inspiration and expiration are worthwhile.

The author has the opinion that this question is more or less academic. Using an incentive spirometer efficiently, the patient has to increase expiration in order to inhale more deeply.

Techniques emphasising expiration like blow-bottle or the inflation of a plastic bag are always proceeded by a very deep inspiration as this is the only way that the patient is enabled to gather the volume need for forced expiration. Once again it is crucial to instruct and train the patient meticulously in order not to compromise him or her.

The aim of all these techniques is an improvement in ventilation and a reduction in mismatches in perfusion.

11.3.1   An Important Point: Coughing

In patients suffering from a pneumothorax with a large air leak it is necessary to eliminate secretions without applying high pressure. An alternative to coughing developed in the UK is "huffing" with an open glottis. This allows the high peak pressures generated while coughing with a closed glottis to be avoided. It is important to bring secretions into the larger airways before huffing in order to suppress the cough reflex for as long as possible. The patient is told to "Puff out towards the mirror"!

In the case of a large air leak, discussion with the physician in charge should be done before initiating the use of an incentive spirometer (Fig. 11.3).

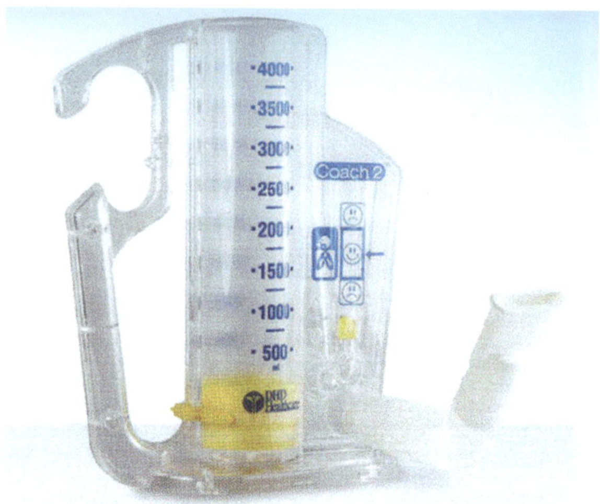

FIGURE 11.3 Incentive spirometer (Coach 2) (Smiths Medical)

Patients suffering from a dry cough are taught to use nasal breathing correctly and moisten their throat (warm drinks etc.). No oral breathing maneuvers should be done during training.

11.4   Dyspnea

Physiotherapists can palliate dyspnea by
- Creating pain free positioning
- Decreasing dyspnea by opening a window or using a fan
- Contact breathing (Fig. 11.4)

Cognition exercises such as "the journey through the body" focus the patient's attention on his body surface to reduce panic and thus optimize breathing by a reflex loop. The physiotherapists Schaarschuch and Haase have developed a concept to optimize perception of one's own body and one's own breathing.

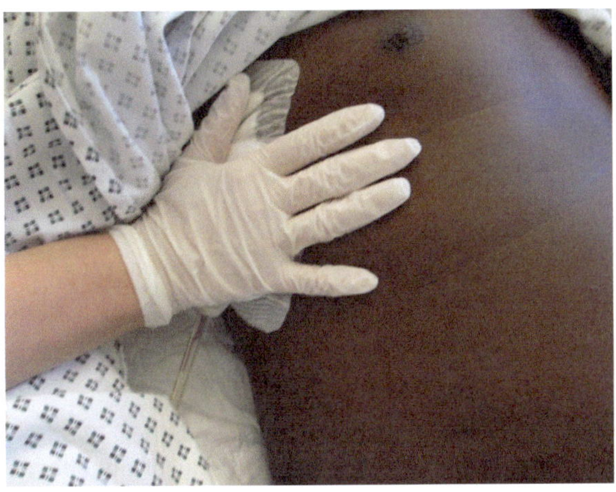

FIGURE 11.4 Contact breathing

11.5 Delirium/Dementia

Delirium and dementia are a challenge for the entire multi-disciplinary team as patients may not be able to participate in sufficient training. In such situation, more creative strategies may be needed to motivate patients, such as turning the therapy into a playful game. Many of these patients have the tendency "to fly out of bed" which can be viewed as a negative but instead could be used with supervision to increase mobilization.

11.5.1 Palliative Care

Palliative care has its own rules which are (re)defined again and again in collaboration with the patient and physiotherapist. The patient may stop or modify therapy whenever wanted. Sometimes family members are included (i.e. in procedures where skin to skin contact is used). The patient's needs are always superior. Creating an atmosphere of confidence is crucial and sometimes just as important as "being there"!

Author's comment:

During my research I mentioned that there are no studies concerning physiotherapy and chest drains. There are no evidence based statements or guidelines concerning this issue. Thus my concept of therapy is pragmatic and functional. In times of limited financial and human resources, it its crucial to identify patients at risk for adverse events early to prevent complications and harm due to chest drain therapy.

Literature

1. Linder A. Thoraxdrainagen und Drainagesysteme. 2014.
2. Arbeitskreis Qi Gong und Medizin. www.qigong-und-medizin.de.
3. Weise S, et al. Empfehlungen zur physiotherapeutischen Atemtherapie. www.atemwegsliga.de.
4. Roth M, Kiefer T. Physiotherapie in der Thoraxchirurgie. 2013.

Chapter 12
Removal of the Chest Drain: How to Do It

Thomas Kiefer

12.1 Criteria for Removal of a Chest Drain

The correct time for removal of a chest drain is mainly determined by two parameters: air leak and fluid production.

12.1.1 Fluid Production

Over the last 20 years, a significant liberalization has taken place in regards to the amount of fluid which should prevent a chest drain from being removed. In the 1970s, chest drainage of less than 100 ml/24 h was required for removal of a chest drain. There have been numerous studies in more recent decades including one from Brunelli et al. [1] that showed that a chest drain in standard thoracic procedures (resections, biopsies, etc) could safely be removed with up to 400 ml/24 h. One study by Bjerregaard et al. [2] demonstrated that a drain could safely be removed with up to 500 ml/24 h of drainage without significant effusion or clinical relevant issue afterward.

T. Kiefer
Chefarzt Klinik für Thoraxchirurgie, Lungenzentrum Bodensee,
Klinikum Konstanz, Luisenstr. 7, 78464 Konstanz, Germany
e-mail: Thomas.Kiefer@glkn.de

© Springer International Publishing Switzerland 2017
T. Kiefer (ed.), *Chest Drains in Daily Clinical Practice*,
DOI 10.1007/978-3-319-32339-8_12

After (talc) pleurodesis, different considerations have to be made. Chest drain outputs below 100 ml/24 h are felt to be sufficiently low to safely remove the drain. It has to be emphasised though that there is no clear evidence for doing so.

After standard procedures, such as lobectomy or segmentectomy, a chest drain can safely be removed with a fluid production of 400 ml/24 h. One must always take into consideration patient specific factors including any underlying disease, the operative procedure, and the quality of the fluid drained.

12.1.2   Air

The second criterion that determines the timing of chest drain removal is the presence of an air leak. If there is no air leak detected and the fluid production is within a tolerable range (see above), the drain(s) can be removed. Experience with electronic drainage systems over many years has shown that small air leaks (20–40 ml/min), which are stable over 6–8 h, are also amenable to safe removal of the chest drain(s) ([3], own experience).

Very small "air leaks" seen with electronic systems can be attributed to their sensitive measurement capabilities. These very small air leaks are clinically irrelevant leaks due to the smallest of leakages in the system (patient – tubing – aggregate).

In such a situation, the observation of a very small stable air leak over a 6–8 h period is crucial before removing the drain.

With the above criteria, a chest drain can be safely removed regardless of how much time has passed since the initial procedure. Unfortunately, there is little information in the literature concerning the correct timing for chest tube removal. Neither the ACCP [4] nor the BTS [5] give any clear recommendations regarding chest tube removal in their very precise and detailed guidelines concerning all other aspects of pneumothorax treatment.

Empyema – whether this is treated by chest drainage alone or in combination with surgery, there is no evidence based data explaining when to remove the drain. The guidelines from the British Thoracic Society [6] are vague for drain removal, and state it can be done "after successful treatment is confirmed radiologically."

Clamping of a chest drain prior to its removal is redundant and can be dangerous. Clamping a chest drain simulates to the body that there is no longer a drain in place. This patient would need to be closely observed and a chest x-ray obtained at a short interval after such a clamping. If the above criteria for chest drain removal are met, the process of clamping is an unnecessary procedure wasting personnel time, resources, and money. It also adds additional radiation exposure albeit low. This maneuver, also has the potential to delay removal of the tube, sometimes for more than a day!

12.1.3   X-Ray Prior to Chest Tube Removal

There is no final or apodictic answer regarding a routine chest x-ray before chest tube removal. Bjerregaard et al. [7] have shown is it safe to avoid a routine chest x-ray prior to removal of a chest drain. Only 10 out of 1097 routine chest x-rays following minimal invasive thoracic surgery (with and without resection) lead to a therapeutic consequence. In my own clinical experience using electronic chest drainage systems, routine chest x-rays were removed from the post procedural protocol safely with the assumed confidence in the electronic system and appropriate patient specific data interpretation.

There is no evidence that in the presence of a patient free of symptoms, a "final" x-ray has to be done – even for medical/legal reasons. In Germany specifically, there is no legal background that forces or justifies doing so.

There is no universally valid scenario as when to remove a chest drain. Each patient should be looked at individually as to the correct time for drain removal based on the procedure done, any underlying disease, and the goal of therapy. In any uncomplicated standard lung resection, the drain can be removed if there is no air leak and fluid production is below the threshold set in that individual center regardless of timing since the procedure.

12.2   Removal of the Chest Drain: Hints on How to Do It

It is well known that patients are very fearful of chest drain removal because of the assumed pain they will have when the drain is removed. Some may have had a previous bad experience with a drain removal from a different area of the body, such as a knee or while it was still on suction. These concerns and fears have to be taken into consideration and the patient has to be reassured.

In the literature there is no consistent recommendation concerning the technique of chest tube removal. The correct way to do so varies greatly from my practice of pulling the drain during breathing arrest in maximal inspiration therefore achieving a maximal pressure in the chest cavity, while others [8] recommend pulling the drain during breathing arrest in maximal expiration having minimal complications. The main complication of concern in this context is a pneumothorax.

After drain removal, a previous placed additional stitch (see Chap. 6 and Fig. 6.8) is secured. An occlusive dressing with povidone-iodine ointment is recommended. Povidone-iodine seals the incision, has a disinfectant affect, and can stop minimal bleeding from the edges of the incision. The ointment is covered by compresses secured with commercially available tape making sure to not make it too tight as skin damage can occur.

A hydrocolloid dressing is an appropriate alternative. This dressing is able to absorb any fluid emanating from the wound.

Imbricated bandages used in earlier days where wound incisions were covered by long overlapping stripes of red paster are obsolete without proven advantage and can be particularly painful at time of removal.

Literature

1. Brunelli A, Beretta E, Cassivi SD, Cerfolio RJ, Detterbeck F, Kiefer T, et al. Consensus definitions to promote an evidence-based approach to management of the pleural space. A collaborative proposal by ESTS, AATS, STS and GTSC. Eur J Cardiothorac Surg. 2011;40(2011):291–7.
2. Bjerregaard LS, Jensen K, Horsleben Petersen R, Hansen HJ. Early chest-tube removal after video-assisted thoracic surgery with serous fluid production p to 500 ml/day. Eur J Cardiothorac Surg. 2014;45:241–6.
3. Linder A. Thoraxdrainagen und Drainagesysteme – Moderne Konzepte. UNI-MED Verlag; 2014.
4. Baumann M, Strange C, Heffner J, et al. Management of spontaneous pneumothorax: an American College of Chest Physicians Delphi consensus statement. Chest. 2001;119:590–602.
5. MacDuff A, Arnold A, Harvey J, on behalf of the BTS Pleural Disease Guideline Group. Management of spontaneous pneumothorax: British Thoracic Society pleural disease guideline 2010. Thorax. 2010;65 Suppl 2:ii18–31.
6. Davies HR, Davies RJO, Davies CWH. Management of pleural infection in adults: British Thoracic Society pleural disease guideline 2010. Thorax. 2010;65:ii41–53. doi:10.1136/thx.2010.137000.
7. Bjerregaard LS, Jensen K, Petersen RH, Hansen HJ. Routinely obtained chest X-rays after elected video-assisted thoracoscopic surgery can be omitted in most patients, a retrospective, observational study. Thorax. 2015;65 Suppl 2:ii18–31.
8. Cerfolio RJ, Bryant AS, Skylizard L, Minnich DJ. Optimal technique for the removal of chest tubes after pulmonary resection. J Thorac Cardiovasc Surg. 2013;145:1535–9.

Index

© Springer International Publishing Switzerland 2017
T. Kiefer (ed.), *Chest Drains in Daily Clinical Practice*,
DOI 10.1007/978-3-319-32339-8

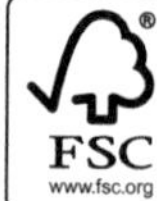